MW00883708

OVARIAN REBOOT

A Personal Journey to Hormone & Fertility *Renewal*

E. Scott Sills

with a *Foreword* by
Samuel H. Wood, MD PhD

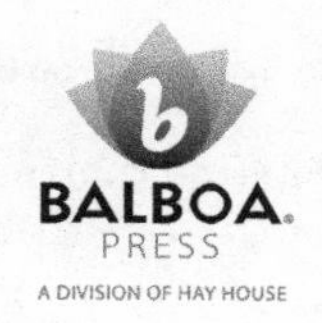

Balboa Press books may be ordered through booksellers or by contacting:

Balboa Press
A Division of Hay House
1663 Liberty Drive
Bloomington, IN 47403
www.balboapress.com
1 (877) 407-4847

Print information available on the last page.

ISBN: 978-1-9822-3214-6 (sc)
ISBN: 978-1-9822-3217-7 (e)

Balboa Press rev. date: 07/27/2019

For my dearest ones
Charles, Ann-Marie, Mary-Kate and Eric,

as well all the wonderful patients
who offered encouragement and support
during difficult times, I remain always grateful.

Contents

Foreword

One of the most challenging problems we encounter as fertility specialists is the progressive loss of fertility which every woman must face. For some, this starts early and results in premature ovarian failure. For others, it arrives later as menopause approaches.

Yet irrespective of age, the struggle to overcome this loss of "ovarian reserve" is real. Finding safe and effective ways to manage this extraordinarily challenging problem has been exceedingly difficult. During seminars at professional conferences, experts have been told for years that "nothing really works," except in the rare case of good fortune.

Against this dreary background, ovarian treatment with a patient's own platelet-derived growth factors has, at last, offered a flash of real hope. This is the so-called *Ovarian Reboot*.

As with many medical interventions, this approach can't always be expected to work for every patient. But we have seen profoundly positive effects for many women, as lost or flagging ovarian function is revived, as the scourge of lost egg quality has, at long last, been overcome, and a healthy child, desired for so very long, is born into the light and hope of life.

Ovarian Reboot recounts the dark history of lost female fertility before the development of ovarian rejuvenation and provides the present status of this remarkable procedure. It brings hope to millions of women who wake up every morning hoping that this month will be different, that this month they will finally achieve their dream of regaining fertility.

And this is just the beginning. Soon, after completing the required scientific research, our team plans to announce Ovarian Regeneration, Generation 2. Although tremendous progress has been made, we still have more to do until all women have the chance to live the hormonal and reproductive life which they desire.

Samuel H. Wood, MD PhD
San Diego, California

"When virtue and modesty enlighten her charms,
the lustre of a beautiful woman is brighter
than the stars of heaven,
and the influence of her power it is in vain to resist."

—Akhenaten (c. 1335 BCE)

One Woman, Her World, and Fertility's Broken Promise

In practical terms, fertility (and how to improve it) is hugely important to the individual woman. It's what keeps IVF clinics open.

But at a more abstract level, it matters for entire populations, too.

Why? We humans had a pitiful population growth rate for thousands of years—less than one tenth of a percent per year! Even now, the typical young couple in the best possible health can expect a monthly pregnancy rate of only around 20%.

The 80% monthly "failure rate" shows that humans are not particularly effective at reproducing.

Anyone who has stood in amazement watching a "world population clock" sees a different story, and knows that count is always changing. The numbers advance fast now, thanks to declines in childhood mortality and whenever mothers have more kids. Of note, human life expectancy has been gaining two to five years each decade since around 1840.

All this happens because babies are born, people migrate, and then we die. And to really understand all these factors, someone needs to measure (or at least estimate) why some women have babies at a young age and some have no kids at all, why some people leave for lands far away to begin a new life while others stay in their hometown, and, of course, why some people die too soon and others reach a very old age.

These factors have been in motion from the beginning, but here we will focus just on the first part, reproduction or fertility—and specifically how the ovary manages that portfolio.

It comes as little comfort to patients having an unsuccessful IVF cycle that we now live in a time of decelerating human fertility. World population growth reached its peak (more than 2%) in the early 1960s and has basically been in a free-fall ever since. Our average fertility rate now hovers near 1.2%; this is expected to be zero by year 2100. And then, population growth for planet Earth will end.

TECHNICAL SNAPSHOT

> The steepest decline in births was among teens between age 15-19, where birth rate dropped 9%. Although teen births are still relatively high in USA compared to some other countries, it has fallen sharply in recent years. This is a trend attributed to greater abstinence and better access to contraception. That decline was slightly offset by more births among women age 40-44, which increased 2%. Births in that older age group has been rising gradually since 1982, most likely due to wider use of more successful advanced reproductive treatments (Sills, 2013; Morrison, 2019).

This is a complex topic, and it's a big ask to portray any one research idea (i.e., ovarian rejuvenation) as a meaningful remedy. But framing the scope of the fertility problem in a macro setting can help see how new "corrections", while not comprehensive, can offer help to one patient at a time. But first, the problem and the suggested approach must be known and fairly appraised.

While nobody books a fertility consult to hear a social studies lecture, some IVF clinics might not see the bigger picture. Does it matter? Well, if you're a patient or a loved one reading this book, at least you have actual data and can form an independent opinion.

When the scope of fertility has been scaled against the world, we can next fix our measure to the individual patient. Yet the journey will draw even closer, to explore the small but essential parts deep inside you, like an engine working quietly in the background. If the ovaries are to be rebooted, or rejuvenated, they first must be appreciated…and then understood.

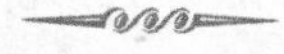

"Memory is the scribe of the soul."

—Aristotle (384–322 BCE)

Your Enigmatic, Essential Essence

From ancient times up to now, there has been one fundamental question about the human condition that always perplexed us: men and women certainly are *not* the same, but why?

What is responsible for these differences? How something so obvious could, at the same time, be so absolutely mysterious continues to draw great interest. And who among us, even today, can fully explain it?

Even before any revered writings or sacred texts were scrolled close to our hearts, every human culture already expressed—and wrestled with—this puzzle. Yes, this same basic theme touches us from prehistoric cave paintings to last week's black-tie classical opera. It remained for scientific research starting in the 1500's to study sex seriously and make meaningful progress.

It remains an important topic to tackle. Originating with the great Hippocrates and later expounded by Galen, there was once a confused belief that some seizures actually happened whenever the womb moved out of the pelvis and pushed upward, into the abdomen or chest. This caused a feeling of 'smothering' which triggered convulsions.

When these ancient writings were rediscovered later in the 14th century, the concept grew to include seizures with any sort of anxiety. This all came to fly under the flag of a condition called 'hysteria'.

It's no coincidence that this term sounds like 'hysterectomy', being closely related to *hysteron*, the Greek name for uterus. Of course, epileptic seizures also happen in people with no womb (men!), but this shortcoming did not stop the great medical thinkers of antiquity. For those cases, bad spirits or demons must surely be the explanation.

Against all this clouded uncertainty, laughing like a riddle within a bigger puzzle, sat the menstrual process itself. Unique to women, this intimate and regular event somehow appeared linked to moon phases and demanded its own answer.

The cycle of fertility was usually predictable and was recognized as absolutely essential for tribal and family structure, because it marked the possibility to conceive and deliver offspring. We call the very first one *menarche,* usually occurring for girls between age 12-15.

But then, for older women who reached sufficient age, something changed here too. Eventually, menstruation stopped. Such females were, sadly, often regarded as barren.

Four hundred years ago, an important clue finally fell into place. The person who discovered the missing piece was Renier de Graaf (1641-1673), a busy Dutch doctor who did considerable research in his spare time.

It is to him that credit is generally given for first identifying the human ovary, its basic parts, and how it might just be the central "timekeeper" which conducts the female fertility orchestra.

While we now understand that the ovary does serve as a skilled conductor, it gets its direction from an even higher authority composing original scores from deep within our brain.

So, in mammals, the harmony of reproduction is attained using a network known as the hypothalamic-pituitary-gonadal (HPG) axis.

This HPG system works like a thermostat or feedback loop, connecting our central nervous system upstairs to 'oversee' the ovaries, lower and much closer to all the action.

This has proven to be a successful way to orchestrate reproduction, dependable over an impressive sweep of evolutionary time.

It's a method which closely mimics what our animal ancestors probably used some 300 million years ago.

It has been proposed that our sex hormones actually reach far outside reproduction. These signals may even act to control how we age, encouraging useful growth early in life but then, in a futile attempt to maintain reproduction later, these same factors work differently—ending up driving the overall ageing process forward.

In this way, one can see how behavior and fate of the ovary should be viewed as so much more than a clutch of oocytes, each egg patiently waiting for an escape each month at ovulation.

But how many know the backstory?

How did the ovary come to be, and how did all those eggs get there in the first place?

I suppose it's a crucial way to frame a challenge, since if our medical aim is to reboot the ovary to some different, stronger, more youthful level of function—even if only temporarily—then we must understand as much as possible about ovarian development and how oocytes (eggs) form in the first place.

If doctors and scientists can deduce *that* pathway, then it becomes possible to change the tempo of ovarian ageing, and thus turn back the biological clock.

"The woman is female, and the man is male; the woman, according to the gynecologist she menstruates or gets sick every month, and the man does not menstruate because he is male."

—M. Gaddafi *The Green Book*, 1975

Difference Confronts Similarity

Our genetic sex is determined at the instant when a particular sperm reaches an egg to fertilize it. Eggs are dependably the same, but there are two types of sperm provided by the man which are available to meet the oocyte.

Depending on whether that sperm carries an X- or Y-chromosome, this is what establishes genetic sex of the resulting embryo—to become a baby approximately 280 days later.

Ways of picking boy or girl offspring have been around as long as anybody can remember, centuries before any of this X or Y chromosome stuff was ever known.

At least two effective techniques remain. Offspring sex may be controlled either by selecting which embryo is put into the womb (by *in vitro* fertilization), or by selecting Y- or X-chromosome bearing sperm (by insemination).

These two methods do involve some medical technology, especially if embryo transfer after IVF is used. But none of the "old wives' tales" you've probably heard of like special diets or sexual positions have ever been found useful to affect genetic sex of offspring.

Getting that X- or Y-chromosome clarified at the moment of fertilization is crucial, because this genetic information (genotype) will be like an architect's blueprint used by nature's construction crew which builds the embryo during gestation.

In fact, during the initial stage of embryo construction inside the womb, each microscopic embryo carries two separate sets of equipment design, male and female—it cannot know just yet which design to follow. This very early period of development is called the "undifferentiated state" and that's okay, there is plenty of time to sort everything out over the next nine months.

But by nine weeks of pregnancy, things are already getting busy. If the fertilizing sperm contributed an X-chromosome, then the genotype will be XX (female).

This means that appropriate embryo tissues will mature into a uterus and fallopian tubes, the structures which reach out to what becomes the ovaries. The genital tubercule develops into the clitoris.

Meanwhile what's needed to build any male equipment simply withers away, since the hormones they need to keep developing are not there (thanks to the absent Y-chromosome).

This sequence sets the stage for a baby girl, her precious ovaries, and the female experience. In the interest of fairness however, the other genetic XY (male) pathway should be covered at least briefly.

If a Y-chromosome (or even a piece of it) is put in the genetic library by the fertilizing sperm, then this triggers production of a certain protein which induces the uncommitted sex gland to make testicles instead of ovaries, and that genital tubercule structure morphs into, you guessed it, a penis.

So in summary, the human female embryo is all set to stay on her track to develop into female form (and, importantly, to shut down all male construction).

Conversely, going down that male pathway won't happen without special signaling. If the Y-chromosome does flag such a detour, this causes a "no-return" exit off the main female turnpike. Most people have heard of one of those decisive hormones, testosterone (the other one is anti-Mullerian hormone, AMH). These two substances are used to make the male embryo turn away from female development, by killing off anything that would make a uterus, cervix, and fallopian tubes.

But let's return to the star of our show, the human ovary. Once the embryo registers no interference from that pesky Y-chromosome and its allies testosterone and AMH, continued progress is possible to develop along the female design.

And by week 12, we are committed either to a female or male (genetic) developmental line. Are there exceptions? Sure. As with much in medicine and surgery practice, there will always be elite cases, but these are complex topics and will need to wait for their own book later.

Yet, continuing with our build-out of the female body from its embryonic beginnings, once any ovarian property starts to be constructed, it really will be of little use if this prime address stays empty. It needs occupants. And what we are leading up to is how the ovary actually gets its eggs, also known more formally as oocytes. So where do *they* come from?

"The world is full of hopeful analogies and handsome, dubious eggs, called possibilities."

—George Eliot (1819-1880)

The Ephemeral Becomes The Eternal

As discussed earlier, learning about the "starts and stops" of the human ovary is essential if we are serious about replicating the process to create new eggs. Figuring out the start point has been the focus of active research.

What is thought to be the oocyte's cellular ancestor—the primordial germ cell (PGC)—shows up very early in embryonic life.

This shows why embryo research has been so useful to map out this complex process. Finally we are beginning to touch some of the missing pieces to this intriguing puzzle. But exactly how they fit into the many empty spaces is proving to be a challenge as well.

What is known now is that in mice, the all-important PGC precursors are seen within the very first week after fertilization. Such precursors develop under the control of special molecular signals, and small clusters of PGCs start appearing along the back of the tiny embryo.

By the time the mouse embryo enters its 12th day after fertilization, most PGCs have already arrived at a place called the genital ridges.

In humans, PGCs are first identified in the yolk sac a bit later than in mice, at the third week of pregnancy. By the time human embryo genital ridges develop by week five, the PGCs have migrated from the hindgut to colonize these structures. And only recently have we been able to fully appreciate the exact steps needed to get from "precursors" to actual eggs that can be fertilized.

Scientists generally agree that getting these PGCs to switch (or differentiate) into eggs is the super critical part, and this step remains the major bottleneck.

So how can this roadblock be managed? Navigating this step is tough. But it's what our research team has been working on, with the generous help of patients willing to assist us. They are the ones who would gain the most from a safe and effective reboot of the ovarian clock, thus enlarging their overall egg pool. And some already have been success stories.

As outlined earlier, in mouse embryos we know these important PGCs develop by the first week after fertilization, and then proliferate up to around 25,000 cells as the second week of embryo development approaches. There exists an intriguing overlap here, between PGCs and primitive steps by the embryo to build other kinds of cells, too.

Being able to form all types of cells in the body (pluripotent), PGCs are important to us because we know that under the right conditions they can absolutely go on to make eggs. Before the second week ends, genital ridge PGCs stop dividing and these egg forerunners enter meiosis, and early eggs (oogonia) are indeed produced next.

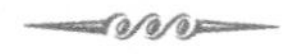

"The pedestal upon which women have
been placed has all too often,
upon closer inspection, been revealed as a cage."

—Ruth Bader Ginsburg (b. 1933)

Unfair Lessons: Sperm Explosion, Egg Extinction

From the viewpoint of the ovary, the pathway ordained for girls is unbelievably different than the one followed by ovary-deficient boys. Even before boys are born, their sperm precursors rush to undergo explosive growth to make spermatogonia, cells which further proliferate and change into an intermediate form called spermatocytes. Next, they become actual sperm.

But what we know now is that there are stem cells in the testicles, too. These cells maintain an amazing ability to self-renew and continue to be active there for the duration of the man's adult life. These are essentially reserve cells, cranking out sperm along with key hormones needed for "maleness".

Could the ovary ever be made to work that renewal trick for eggs?

Like much in reproductive science, this area can stir controversy. Some experts claim that primordial germ cells are actually not present in the testes, disappearing from both testicles *and* ovaries by adulthood.

But, wait. We know something *has* to be different for men to keep their sperm production active essentially for their entire life.

These divergent views might be explained by different ways laboratories mark (or label) specific cells, hence the confusion. Yet even the dissenters agree that there is a special group of cells with the ability to renew, mixed in with ovarian and testicular tissue.

On the development highway, could these cells really be those essential PGCs, incognito and somehow existing unseen in the ovary?

These are important players. In the adult ovary, there is another possibly different group of very small embryonic-like stem cells and go by another abbreviation, VSELs. These VSELs draw little dispute among experts and are definitely present in adult ovaries. VSELs don't seem to do much, possibly explaining why they were under our radar and remained undetected for so long.

These quiet cells have some interesting properties, like being tough customers able to sustain radiation and stay functional in older, non-functional ovaries. Their ability to act like the female "reserve cell" is shown by the VSELs capacity to self-renew and grow into a variety of other tissue types.

Discovery of such a feature, again, would be of tremendous benefit to fertility patients since under correct management this could lead to the growth of new oocytes. Thus far, the wide developmental potential in VSELs has been experimentally confirmed in both mice and humans.

So, whether we call these cells with apparently "rejuvenating" powers as PGCs or VSELs, it may not matter much. Any controversy may come from honest differences in how various labs label cells in an area where, admittedly, there has not been much standardization yet.

Such similarities notwithstanding, there are some differences between migrating PGCs (size = 15–20 μm) and VSELs (size = 3-6 μm). More research is needed to determine if VSELs are more developmentally primitive than PGCs. PGCs may be a precursor to pluripotent stem cells in vitro, although they do not seem to behave as stem cells *in vivo.* Indeed, later in male fetal development the true stem cell population appears in the testis and divides throughout life, yielding ongoing sperm production. The ovary could have comparable cells with stem-like characteristics, capable of differentiating into eggs.

This is new territory and while important work continues, perhaps the advancement with the most significant impact for fertility care is this: Whatever we may call them, there are cells in the adult ovary that, with proper treatment, seem to have a capacity to produce new eggs.

If VSELs are indeed functionally and developmentally equivalent to PGCs as precursors to eggs, then as long as it's safe, most patients won't really care what abbreviation is used to tag them. Who knows, maybe VSELs might be the same thing as PGCs, or their precursors.

Anything with the ability to help make new eggs is worth studying, right?

And science has already proved that VSELs can spontaneously do this, *if given the right signals*. Other cells known as mesenchymal cells can be put inside the ovary and restore reproductive function. Those extra cells are added to the lab dish to support and nurse the VSELs. Amazingly, this approach already has been used successfully to produce a livebirth in a woman who had premature ovarian failure.

What we need to know next is how to harness this power, to be applied for anyone with ovaries needing a reboot.

"Somewhere, something incredible
is waiting to be known."

—Carl Sagan (1934-1996)

Somewhere, Ovary Rainbow

As already discussed, the most important jobs of the ovary are to sustain egg development and to make the hormones needed to be female. Without these steps, fertility fails.

The task includes launching puberty at the right time. It's true, the ovary essentially runs the human reproductive cycle (and pregnancy) over the entire reproductive career of a woman.

To do this, all the interlocking functions need a constant cascade of remodeling and regression. This requires a lot of biochemical and tissue coordination.

Of note, several ovarian disorders like polycystic ovary syndrome, premature ovarian insufficiency/failure, and even ovarian cancer have all been linked with disturbances in how certain cells behave within the ovary.

Newer research has suggested ways to boost ovarian response during fertility treatments, including IVF. Some of this work will be reviewed here later, but even with all our experimental work, more questions have emerged as findings from early studies are assessed.

In the meantime, any effort to enhance or extend fertility will come from the best possible knowledge of the cell and tissue remodeling processes in the ovary. Sharing such information and putting it all in one place is one of the reasons this book exists.

Although we can understand much about ovarian development using "comparative anatomy" and related structures (particularly the adrenal gland and testis), there are limits to what can be applied to the ovary when looking at these other organs.

Can you think of something that sets the human ovary apart from all other organs? Ovaries are indeed special, but one characteristic makes them unlike any other female endocrine organ: The ovary undergoes massive, extensive, re-wiring when puberty hits.

Even during early embryo growth, the mechanism for ovary formation is elegant and far from simple. As a derivative of the "noncommitted" early tissue ready to switch either to male or female, the ovary must transit past that brief phase where the potential for each sex exists. Yet, some parts of the ovary actually arrive from other sources, like an import.

While the ovary itself is still in its embryonic stages, this list of "guest" cells checking in actually includes the very cells that will eventually develop into what we are most interested in—eggs.

These egg precursors are of course critically important in fertility medicine, although not many women may know that they actually start from outside the ovary, coming from a structure called the yolk sac.

As these proto-oocytes journey into their designated niche within the ovary, a lot of interplay happens among all the cells they meet along the way. Indeed, the crosstalk of molecular signals between these early eggs and other cells of the ovary appears critical. In other words, the way the ovary is built out appears to be influenced by the egg itself, as if oocytes help to ensure that their neighborhood is fully committed to female anatomy.

This allows tiny structures called "primordial follicles" to develop from what continues to stream into the ovary. Once this recruitment is done, these small spheres grow through primary, preantral, antral, and preovulatory stages before full maturation, and then release an egg at ovulation.

Oocytes also control the cells which most closely surround them (called granulosa cells), stopping any interference with egg release, like disordered or premature growth.

Running parallel to this mutually beneficial dialogue between eggs and other nearby ovarian cells, evidence now exists to show that some pre-eggs (germ cells) are present on or near the ovarian surface. Interestingly, when the embryonic ovary finally finishes developing and its capsule closes, the once "open" partitions inside it close too.

As the ovary zips up this surface tissue sheet, some egg precursors can get marooned up at the ovarian surface. But why? What evolutionary advantage may be gained from it?

Neither the purpose nor function of these stranded germ cells (egg precursors) at the ovarian surface are known, but they have attracted outsized importance. Their presence has big implications for natural hormone recovery and fertility potential.

Why? Because these cells may be the source of germline stem cells, parked inside adult ovaries. These are cells that are able to become new oocytes. And the reason these cells matter now is that, at least for past half century, doctors and patients have both just assumed that the entire number of eggs is fixed at birth.

Our accepted, traditional way of thinking is a concept you may remember from high school biology. It goes something like this: Human ovaries are not supposed to have a way to put any deposits into this "egg account".

Sadly, from this egg endowment, only withdrawals are possible until the balance gradually runs down over time, reaching zero at menopause.

And here is where things turn especially interesting. The traditional concept of ovarian reserve met a challenge in 2004, sparking a debate. What if these "special cells" tucked away at the ovary surface were the true source of new eggs?

To everyone's great surprise, putative germline stem cells (stem cells which can turn into new eggs) were indeed discovered in ovaries of adult humans. But how could this be? Perhaps there was a mistake. It just had to be an error, because if true, it would mean revamping one of the most important concepts in human biology.

Other laboratories reported the same thing in other mammals where biological clocks run too, including mice and rats. In fact, the first description of germ cells in postnatal mice ovaries was reported after examining changes in follicle numbers over time.

These investigators later saw expression of germline markers in cells taken from the bone marrow. Interestingly, bone marrow transplants allowed recovery of some egg production in mice that had been intentionally sterilized by chemotherapy—something which should have killed all the eggs, making the mice permanently sterile.

From this, scientists thought that bone marrow might be a potential source of female germ cells. But additional studies failed to confirm this approach as a workable option. Thus far, there have not been any women who achieved pregnancy from stem cell injections into their ovaries.

Getting any new eggs to appear for subsequent harvest and fertility treatment was turning out to be a bit more difficult than first imagined. It was back to the drawing board, where one key question lingered without a satisfactory answer.

It seemed unlikely that eggs originate from a bone marrow stem cell source. Prior experiments proved that. This dead-end was further confirmed by "molecular clock" experiments, which tried to estimate the number of divisions over a cell's entire lifetime.

Curiously, what we learned was there was an assembly-line model of egg development at work, where the earliest oocytes eligible for ovulation are also the first eggs to get ready for ovulation. This study turned up some useful information about egg design, but really didn't add much to where they—or their precursors—might originate.

But then, something exciting was reported when a population of mitotically active cells in adult mouse ovaries were successfully tweaked to show some germline characteristics. Remembering that getting germline features was the key step to make new eggs from scratch (*de novo*), many scientists wanted to take a closer look at this fascinating twist.

The work was recognized as pathbreaking, and as usual much was challenged by other experts. This was because it could not be absolutely verified that such cells really could be made to produce fresh eggs (postnatal oogenesis). Not willing to let go of this opportunity so fast, others built on this idea with a clever experiment.

They used a transplantation model to repopulate cells in mouse ovaries which were first hit with powerful chemo, it was shown that cells consistent with ovarian germline stem cells (the building blocks needed to build *de novo* eggs) were still there.

But where in the ovary could they be found? Sophisticated labelling studies were next pressed into service to crack the case.

From this, it was thought that the ovary capsule (epithelium) was the source of germline stem cells. Some experts in developmental anatomy and embryology weren't surprised by reports that ovarian stem cells might be just under the "skin" of adult ovaries.

More success soon followed. Those germline stem cells were proved to be correctly identified based on surface markers only found in stem cells, and then were used to produce healthy baby mice.

Still using a mouse model, researchers were able to achieve a major jump start on fertility. They showed that if they could get a particular kind of stem cell from the ovary, which had now been proven to exist, then that cell could be "processed" (matured) up to a level close enough to a regular egg and be successfully fertilized. Moreover, such a fertilized egg could be grown to an embryo stage far along enough to transfer it to a recipient adult mouse...where it could grow and be born later.

While this was certainly big news, caution was still urged from the researchers most familiar with this high-tech method of mouse making.

The reason people hesitated was the disappointingly low efficiency in converting such cells into eggs. It could be done, but there needed to be a way to increase effectiveness for things to get serious.

While less than 1% of "seeded" germline stem cells spontaneously turned into oocyte-like cells, this oocyte conversion yield was enhanced when certain factors were added to the mix.

Given the importance of these findings, it was not entirely surprising that other researchers hopped on the bandwagon and began to criticize the whole experiment, especially the lab protocol used to make any new eggs.

That's how science needs to work, by getting input from experts who love to shoot down results with keen observations of their own. If that criticism is used to improve study design, we can advance.

Better cell labeling was suggested to isolate and purify germline stem cells, and this lined up with earlier work finding that primitive germ cells could indeed make fertilizable oocytes—and later embryos.

Of course, eventually it was time to apply these mouse results to something more useful in doctors' offices. Encouragingly, germline stem cells were indeed obtained from adult human ovaries and cultured in a controlled lab setting.

When these cells were put deep into human ovaries, sure enough, they soon developed into what looked like early eggs (and this was double-checked with gene marker labeling). These inserted cells later even found themselves surrounded by granulosa cells to form follicles just like regular eggs.

This is the kind of activity completely lacking in the impaired ovary, when the supply of functional follicles and eggs is totally exhausted. Those key cells are gone and are not coming back, and this is the enemy. This is menopause.

TECHNICAL SNAPSHOT

Disagreement exists on the preferred technique to isolate germline stem cells. Relying on Ddx4/MVH expression to isolate and purify

> germline stem cells is problematic, since Ddx4 (a type of RNA helicase) can also be present in germ cell cytoplasm (Castrillon *et al,* 2000). It appears that "immature" germline cells are present in the ovary, capable of expressing Ddx4 or domains of Ddx4 on the cell surface. After development is locked down the oocyte pathway, Ddx4 goes away and is no longer externally expressed (Imudia *et al,* 2013).

Other methods to identify and isolate germline stem cells in mice with improved efficiency with antibodies and antibody-assisted magnetic-bead sorting have also been used.

Encouraging for our story, female germline stem cells from mice can be changed into pluripotent embryonic stem-like cells in the right environment. Of note, such germline stem cells display similar features as male germline stem cells and sperm precursors.

When researchers reported that, it was like finally discovering the key to a long-locked door…behind which lies the secret to ovarian rejuvenation.

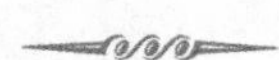

"Into her womb
convey sterility.
Dry up in her
the organs of increase."

—King Lear; Act I, Scene 4

Unpacking Menopause

A woman in menopause will, most likely, now end up living a long time after her ovaries quit working, usually decades after her last successful pregnancy (if there ever was one). But what exactly is this last stop on the ovarian train track? And why is it even here?

Menopause is rarely welcomed. Often its symptoms arrive way too soon and with no notice, drastically damaging fertility prospects. Biologists consider this to be the "post-reproductive" phase of female life. But maybe we should feel special, because very few animals even experience it!

Experts agree that this thing called menopause is remarkable across the entire animal kingdom. It is actually limited to us humans and just a few types of toothed whales.

As our life expectancy increases with better overall health and modern medical care, this means there are more menopausal females at any given time. And the low birth rate in USA (as discussed before) tells us that the young females who are best able to reproduce are not doing so.

This leads us to perhaps the most fundamental (yet least discussed) principles in primary care medicine: The chief predictor of reproductive success is the age of the woman.

Some fertility patients dream of getting pregnant and say "I may be 47, but everybody tells me I only look 30 and I certainly do feel young!" In denial, the fact that careful assessment shows that they probably ran out of eggs long before today's consult is simply ignored.

This is a truly sad situation, and deeply unfair to those who are otherwise in perfect health. But all this really shows is that women have successfully "uncoupled" reproductive function from everything else their bodies can still do amazingly well, often into advanced age.

But from where our IVF patients stand, this doesn't make much sense.

After all, wouldn't it be better for humans to maximize our evolutionary fitness, to hold on to reproduce capacity right up until the end of life? Get pregnant whenever you want, irrespective of age!

While this aspiration won't appeal to every woman, it resonates strongly for some. But biology needs more than your wish list to be persuaded. For females the ability to attain a pregnancy starts to get depressingly blunted around age 35.

The reason ovarian reserve drops so soon, and is eventually shadowed by menopause, may never be known. If non-functioning ovaries with no more eggs are so common, then what can possibly be the reason?

It's a highly relevant issue for you who may want a baby of your own, and as covered from the start, for entire populations of nations who must remain demographically viable. At first glimpse, it does seem to be a tragic waste. Is there no redeeming feature that can be attributed to menopause?

Possibly, yes.

We know from field studies that limited food sharing is seen between parent and offspring in many primates. But only among humans do mothers provide most of their weaned children's dietary needs. This allows mothers to use resources that they themselves can apply at high efficiency, but that their baby cannot.

For example, some hunter–gatherer groups use deeply buried roots as a year-round food source. Our babies can't do much with that by themselves, but their moms are skilled enough to find that food surplus, often getting enough so that more than one child can survive. Of course, any older women past menopause can earn the same high rates of food collection.

In this social model, while menopause may not be useful or beneficial to a specific female, it can nevertheless contribute to tribe or family survival overall.

With no young children of their own, such females who can't or won't get pregnant (again) could still help support their daughters' or nieces' offspring.

So back when we were cave dwellers, it was apparently a good thing to have an Aunt or Grandmother who had no cubs of her own…but still looked after us when we were very little.

Especially for the nutritional welfare of any weaned children, this contribution by older women is crucial when mothers forage less when another baby arrives on the scene.

If this theory about menopause is right, then childbearing women should produce babies faster because of (post-fertility) grandmothers' indirect contribution to production.

From prehistoric times, this "It Takes a Village" approach seems to give a workable answer to the mystery of menopause in humans. Our close primate relatives usually live no longer than about 50 years. That is, the rest of their body ages much faster than ours, so that all primate life functions, including fertility, usually fail at about the same time.

For us, maximum lifespan occasionally reaches 100 years (sometimes even more) and although fertility in women is spent well before half that time, this is still well in advance of most other aspects of physiological frailty.

The question is how natural selection came to favor this distinctly human post-reproductive component of life history. It's worth considering that this Grandmother Hypothesis is the answer.

"Though the sex to which I belong
is considered weak,
you will nevertheless find me
a rock that bends to no wind."

—Elizabeth I (1533-1603)

Nature's Building Blocks

Remember the way an early embryo goes about recruiting building blocks for eggs? Those early cells migrated and arrived in the right place at the right time. The developing ovary received its compliment of oocytes, like an egg endowment.

Our story picks up here, as either PGCs or VSELs are now thought to be those very primordial germ cells which move into the forming ovary. The interesting thing now is that they are thought to persist long into adulthood.

The developing ovary can be thought of as an anatomical starter house, the best possible place an egg can live. Although individual eggs can't be seen on office ultrasound equipment, as any IVF patient will know, follicles can usually be detected and measured this way.

Starting with a primordial follicle, it takes about 150 days for things to grow up to the next (preantral) stage and then another 120 days after that to build each antral follicle (secondary).

This is the point where most fertility shots get a chance to work their magic. But if the antral follicle count is low (or zero), then it's no big surprise that nothing much can happen with IVF treatment—no matter the medication dose. This is the most common reason IVF cycles are cancelled for "poor response".

In younger women who do IVF, a cohort of antral follicles will hopefully respond over some 10-15 days to mature, and then be surgically retrieved and prepared for fertilization. Whether or not an antral follicle pool is big enough to work with can now be estimated by *ovarian reserve screening.*

Measuring anti-Mullerian hormone (AMH) is done by a blood test and is often used to check a woman's ovarian reserve well before IVF is even booked. Understandably, a fertility center wouldn't encourage anyone to start a major procedure if the egg tank is already empty.

This AMH test is worth knowing more about, especially for anybody contemplating doing an IVF cycle. Fertility clinics rely on this blood test a lot, to predict how well a woman might react to fertility medications used to get many eggs.

Thus, AMH can be thought of like a gas gauge on your egg tank. Anyone serious about trying IVF really should, at some point, ask for this blood test.

Notwithstanding any controversies of the AMH blood test as a fertility predictor, its common use as a gatekeeper in egg donation tends to support picking it as a reliable benchmark for anyone's personal egg supply.

Should you be lucky enough to have a high AMH number, then your ovaries probably still have many eggs available.

And if the AMH level is low or zero, you might find many clinics don't return your call. They already know you've got nothing to work with, so why bother? As you might expect, when menopause hits, AMH is basically undetectable.

If you accept that serum AMH level can work like a "proxy marker" for egg reserve, then this might be a good way to confirm a change in ovarian function following some treatment. If the AMH goes up afterward, this would be a good sign.

And if you are persuaded that adult ovaries have special egg precursors that, when switched on, can make new eggs (where

AMH can climb out of the basement) then…all that's missing is some way to reach in there and hit the proper switch to make it happen.

But has this ever been done, and, if yes, how might it work?

"You never change things by fighting the existing reality.
To change something, build a new model
that makes the existing model obsolete."

—Buckminster Fuller (1895-1983)

Personally Recapturing Possibilities

If a scientist wanted to find a dependable pack of cellular growth signals, not synthesized in a lab or by drug companies but made organically by the patient herself—which could then be used to awaken the adult ovary—then platelet rich plasma (PRP) would be a good place to look first.

This is because PRP already has been used effectively to treat other tissue disorders. We know it is safe. PRP is comprised of molecules which coordinate cellular repair after tissue injury.

Closely linked to the same signals involved when tissue is inflamed, PRP figures prominently in regenerating tissue, cell proliferation, extracellular matrix remodeling, shutting off certain cells by "programmed cell death", differentiation, and growing new blood vessels.

Think of platelets as a type of biological envelope, and this sealed packet is crammed full of letters (cell signals) which, when opened and read by the target (ovary), messages get delivered instructing the nearby cells to do specific things.

Now consider what happens each month on the ovary surface, when a mature egg pops out at ovulation. Even though we take it for granted, there is actually considerable wear and tear on the ovary every time its lining gets a tiny hole in it. How does the ovary fix that surface spot where ovulation just happened?

It's already known that PRP plays a role in the local tissue repair response following ovarian epithelial microtrauma after ovulation, and it probably helps with overall ovary function too. But the effects of PRP and its associated growth factors in the ovaries were not given much thought until lately.

How could this be explored more carefully?

In 2017, a study was launched here to look at this issue. There was a suspicion that PRP was doing something to the ovary, and even before patient enrollment closed, there were reports suggesting that intraovarian application of PRP could lift ovarian reserve, allow eggs to be collected, and build embryos. In the meantime, early results from similar PRP techniques started to show up in peer-review medical journals.

The registered clinical trial gathered lab data from 182 women who completed ovarian PRP and then underwent monitoring. While serum FSH, E_2, and AMH were each checked over time, the latter was classified as the primary marker of ovarian reserve, given the relative consistency of AMH throughout the menstrual cycle.

The average age for the females in this group was just over 45, and most had already failed IVF before. Some had already stopped having menstrual cycles anyway, so serum AMH is preferred in this setting where there is no "cycle day".

To simplify analysis of what happened next, patient responses to intraovarian PRP were put into one of two groups. Better ovarian reserve (increase in serum AMH vs. baseline) was called "Category A". Alternatively, if there was no change/decrease seen in AMH then this was termed "Category B".

All patients tolerated the ovarian PRP injection well; the procedure was performed in an IVF office under ultrasound guidance. It took about 10 minutes an no anesthesia was needed; there were no complications.

It turned out that putting PRP into ovarian tissue led to better fertility potential in just under 30% of cases. Specifically, the desirable improvement 'Category A' response accounted for 28% of the study group, while 72% of women showed no AMH gain after treatment as 'Category B'.

But what made ovarian PRP work for some women, but not others? The search was on to find out if anything could predict this.

Patient weight did not seem to matter, as average BMI was not that different among patients, no matter how their AMH behaved. However, women with the top BMI value in Category A and B were around 33 and 46, respectively, so the non-responders *were* a bit heavier.

So if body mass index couldn't predict response vs. non-response, what other factors might explain the observed results?

It was first thought that any of the high post-treatment AMH levels we saw after PRP (suggesting improved fertility potential) might be attainable only among younger females. It was crucial to check this idea, because a bit more than 25% of study patients were less than 42 years old.

If younger women were the only patients who responded to ovarian PRP, then this would suggest that, when it comes to ovarian PRP therapy, older women shouldn't bother with it.

Interestingly, when all patient data were broken down and put into categories by age (women younger than age 42 compared to patients age 42 and up), both groups showed significant gains in serum AMH after treatment.

In fact, the average AMH lift was actually *better* for older women who received ovarian PRP, although this was probably due how statistics gives more weight to larger sample sizes.

A few other areas were examined as well, including if one or both ovaries received the PRP shot.

All women entered the study expecting that both ovaries would get freshly prepared PRP. This was always our goal, too. But injecting PRP into both sides safely was impossible for some women. This "unilateral ovarian injection" usually was an issue when one ovary couldn't be seen clearly on internal (transvaginal) ultrasound—something more common among heavier women.

But placement of PRP in just one ovary didn't hold back the helpful lift in AMH seen after treatment. This suggested that although injecting PRP into both ovaries may be nice to aim for, it doesn't seem to be a deal-breaker. We confirmed this when the percentage of "one ovary only" cases was counted in the two patient response groups, and there was no statistically important difference noted.

In other words, if placing platelet-derived growth factors in both ovaries really was super necessary to see desirable increases in AMH levels later, then we would expect to see a big cluster of "one ovary only" cases in Category B—women who showed no benefit in ovarian reserve after PRP injection.

But this wasn't what was found.

Finally, we examined the platelet count right before PRP was injected into the ovaries. This was done because, after all, the first 'P' in PRP stands for platelets!

The thinking was that maybe women with higher platelet numbers might somehow fare better when PRP was put into their ovarian tissue.

Sure enough, average baseline platelet levels for Category A and B patients did show a big difference. Our "good responder" (Category A) cases had mean platelet counts significantly higher compared to women who didn't show an AMH improvement—A vs. B was 274K and 250K, respectively.

In my view, the discovery that a woman's platelet count somehow relates to the AMH response after intraovarian PRP treatment is notable. And in retrospect, it made sense.

This observation argues against the belief that simply sticking a needle into the ovary (sham injection or "ovarian acupuncture") is all that's required for a meaningful AMH change.

If that was right, then no matter what the platelet situation was, the AMH reaction would be the same because the crucial event would be the injection itself—not what substance was being placed into the ovary. The work from the clinical trial offers a new look at this very intriguing process, and what can be possible when PRP is used in a standardized way.

But so what if AMH goes up after PRP is injected into the ovaries? If you want a baby, having a blood test showing a better AMH level is a long way from sending out birth announcements.

This would be a fair critique. It must be admitted that while elevated AMH after using this PRP protocol would be a desirable result for older women with previously low reserve, it's not the same as a healthy term livebirth.

So even though this was the first research to look at AMH response to a standard protocol of PRP samples being injected into ovarian tissue, repairing low reserve is a small step on a long journey. It's also true that ovarian PRP does not work for every patient.

Yet it's worth remembering that the IVF process can never get off the ground without eggs. And serum AMH is the best upstream marker that we have to predict if those eggs can be harvested. It also has been shown that while the ovary is trying to switch back on and build new eggs, the hormonal situation it orchestrates is changing in unexpected ways even before any eggs arrive.

Making more eggs for those who need them is wonderful, assuming those eggs are good enough to use. But can anything be done if this is not the case?

"Make the most of your regrets; never smother your sorrow,
but tend and cherish it till it comes to have
a separate and integral interest.
To regret deeply is to live afresh."

—Henry David Thoreau (1817-1862)

When More Isn't Better

The information we can get from AMH testing is good, but it's not perfect. AMH is all about estimating the *number* of eggs potentially available in the ovary, something that's critical to know before beginning any fertility treatment.

Although serum AMH does well in predicting ovarian reserve, it tells us nothing about egg *quality*.

In fact, at this stage we don't really have any way to tell this. There is no common, reliable way to find out anything about oocyte quality until the egg is taken out with an attempt to fertilize it. And that means doing an IVF cycle.

In other words, a patient could have more than one problem. She may have a low number of eggs, and any eggs that she does have may also be of very low quality.

One reason why multiple IVF cycles keep failing is that the only thing that usually changes, one treatment to the next, are minor adjustments to the fertility medications used. But when it comes to egg quality, it's now believed that IVF shots arrive far too late to make much difference.

Embryo development actually begins much earlier, during the time when eggs and their precursors are still developing in the ovary. From earlier chapters here, this concept should be familiar.

Thus, if we want to improve the integrity of the egg, attention should be focused considerably upstream, well before when follicles are recruited in IVF.

This is something many older IVF patients routinely face. The problem of genetic imbalance in the embryo (a condition called aneuploidy) is an unwelcome and serious detour on the road to pregnancy. It means the embryo is not genetically normal, and such embryos generally are not used and treatment stops.

Developing a way to enhance chromosomal competency of embryos is a long-sought goal of fertility doctors. This would be a discovery with an impact difficult to overstate, if it could be done.

In 2019, a medical paper was published showing how platelet-derived growth factors could be successfully used before IVF, for this exact purpose.

The case was unusual. This patient was a healthy 42-year old. She and her partner had struggled with infertility for three years. By the time I met them, five cycles of IVF had already happened—they had produced 20 embryos, but sadly, all had genetic abnormalities. No embryo transfer was ever done.

No reason for this could be found, as every lab test was completely normal.

It was beginning to be known that our group was using ovarian PRP to increase egg number, but what was not known was the result PRP might have on egg quality. This patient asked if ovarian PRP might help her get better eggs, not simply more of them. We agreed to find out.

Prior to IVF here, she received two injections (some three months apart) of platelet-derived growth factors injected into both ovaries. She later completed an IVF and made one genetically normal boy embryo, which was frozen at the blastocyst stage.

Nine days after thaw and transfer, she got a positive pregnancy test. Ultrasound scan at six weeks' gestation confirmed a single intrauterine pregnancy with a strong heart rate at 153 beats per minute.

From this, it was inferred that intraovarian application of platelet-derived growth factors, when used before IVF, can help improve egg quality and make genetically normal embryos possible.

Although research on intraovarian injection of PRP had already shown improved quantitative IVF responses, this was the first finding of improved embryo genetics after intraovarian injection of autologous platelet-derived growth factors.

Lessons from this case give a new way to tackle the previously hopeless question "What can be done to repair any genetic problems with my embryos?"

Like much in IVF practice, the precise way growth factors from platelets might impact chromosomal competency during oogenesis remains speculative.

It has already been shown that platelets release cytokines, chemokines, and growth factors including platelet-derived growth factor (PDGF), stromal cell derived factor 1 (SDF-1) and hepatocyte growth factor (HGF)—many vital letters inside an important envelope.

These molecular signals push the right buttons for recruitment, proliferation, and activation of fibroblasts, neutrophils, monocytes and many other cells. This part is known from an accumulation of many published studies.

And when those signals get to the ovary, these mediators likewise would be expected to amplify new blood vessel growth providing better tissue perfusion. So raising the oxygen level inside the ovary (attained when new capillaries are in service) is just one way improvement in egg genetics might happen after PRP treatment.

But how? Placing PRP cytokines into ovarian tissue may cause higher AMH and improved blastocyst genetics—and both have now been reported—in at least two ways.

One mechanism is that any follicles recruited (and oocytes obtained) after intraovarian injection of these growth factors were really there to begin with—sleepy, but then stimulated. On the other hand, upon contacting ovarian tissue these platelet growth factors engaged with uncommitted VSELs and/or PGCs, supplying molecular signals needed to promote differentiation to develop *de novo* eggs.

Scientists have recently proved that PRP helps growth and survival of isolated early human follicles in lab studies. When cells are incubated with PRP-supplemented culture media, they grow significantly better than when this supplementation is lacking.

It is also known that older women make eggs with fewer mitochondria. This little organ is the powerplant of the cell. Older eggs also have impaired fertilization, and poor embryonic development, all possibly due to altered mitochondria.

A strong connection here seems plausible, as relatively high levels of mitochondrial DNA has been reported among genetically abnormal embryos. In other words, the cell knows it suffers from a growth crisis, so it tries to compensate for this by cranking out more batteries (mitochondria). If one result of ovarian treatment with PRP is simply improved ooplasm quality, then a subsequent mitochondrial reset is another process by which ploidy rescue of blastocysts might operate.

More research is needed to build on this compelling story. Replenishment of eggs is always good. But getting better *quality* oocytes (and embryos) as shown here, is much better.

"We are always the same age inside."

—Gertrude Stein (1874-1946)

There is Life Beyond Fertility

When periods begin to get irregular, this heralds the natural closing of the reproductive window for women.

The effects of this narrowing therapeutic spectrum in clinical fertility practice may be regarded as universal among women of sufficient age, to impact productivity and quality of life with much variation.

Indeed some women may not confront menopause until quite old, but nevertheless they can experience some features of ovarian ageing. Reproductive loss is just one component.

Of course fertility issues will usually take the spotlight during my IVF consultations, but not far from centerstage are equally distressing issues which may not get talked about.

These changes might include vaginal discomfort and dryness, reduced sex drive, not sleeping well, and "brain fog" or cognitive decline.

Estradiol and testosterone are both made in the ovary and, independent of trying to get pregnant, these sex hormones absolutely shape the overall female experience.

But what if pregnancy isn't the goal? For such patients, the way injection of PRP into the ovary might change sexual or neurobehavioral response could still be useful.

It has recently been shown that major increases in sexual activity, better ability to reach orgasm/climax, and elevated overall sexual experience were reported by women who had ovarian PRP injection here.

Very few sources are aware of these new data, and you can bet that the pharmaceutical industry would be perfectly delighted to keep it that way.

How might the dramatic changes observed here be explained? What is it about injecting autologous PRP into impaired or dormant ovarian tissue that could yield an apparent alteration in function?

Discussion of IVF cycle data after ovarian PRP permitted some guesswork. We already know that placing PRP inside ovarian tissue delivers growth factors, chemokines, and cytokines like stromal cell derived factor-1, hepatocyte growth factor, and maybe dozens of others, deep into that target.

Upon arrival, these molecular signals orchestrate tissue perfusion and angiogenesis clearing the way for ovarian re-potentiation.

Indeed, placement of PRP in the proper place seems to "switch on" adult ovaries with low or absent reserve. This explains why the AMH can go up after PRP injection and getting any eggs might only be a secondary reaction. Growth factors seem to set up a two-stage process, follicles as a foundation first, followed by eggs (hopefully) arriving later.

In other words, by establishing communication channels with uncommitted ovarian stem cells, this creates local signaling contexts leading to differentiation towards hormonally active follicles.

Higher levels of hormone output from the ovaries may have been triggered by all those platelet-derived growth factors. It's possible that when those molecules arrived and pushed the right buttons in "tired" ovarian tissue, endocrine function was restored to younger levels.

In other words, a kind of PRP "rescue" may have happened. This could be why many of our 80 study patients had big improvements across a range of areas, including sleep quality, energy level, better nail strength, skin texture, scalp hair growth, clarity of thinking, as well as "wetter" cervical mucus production and vaginal lubrication.

At least one woman celebrated by updating her wardrobe. She told the tale of getting some "nice black boots" after her PRP procedure. According to her, this victory purchase had not been seen in her closet for many years. The story even helped influence the cover image for this book!

So yes, these "quality of life" issues did get much better following use of intraovarian PRP, even if the woman wasn't seeking fertility treatments. We know this could matter to a huge female population: These patients are not interested in pregnancy, they just want their life back.

Since none of these women were taking any hormone pills, estrogen patches or creams, the effects reported on their anonymous, confidential questionnaires must have been linked to something that was drastically altered in their "rejuvenated" ovaries. Nothing else had changed.

One unexpected finding in this study came from an analysis of patient age and whether or not that influenced the woman's response after ovarian PRP treatment.

We discovered that improved overall sexual experience was noted by older women, a result that certainly invites more study. This observation suggests that ovaries in older women may actually be better suited for ovarian PRP.

Based on the sweeping scope of changes reported by these women, should ovarian PRP be considered for those who suffer from menopausal issues, even if they do not want fertility treatment and don't care about retrieving their own eggs?

This question is key because a growing body of evidence is now available on the health of older women. Usually this carries an emphasis on exercise, diet, toxin avoidance, and especially hormone replacement. That last listing powers a multi-billion dollar industry.

Because symptoms of menopause can be severe and sometimes don't respond to common prescription drugs, doctors often deploy multiple strategies at the same time. Yet there are always cases where medication side effects are too severe, or the treatment simply fails.

It would be a happy forecast if ovarian PRP could help these patients. If early results with ovarian PRP can be validated by additional multi-center studies, then using PRP in this way could join the existing, conventional treatments for menopausal symptoms.

While it is certainly far too soon to consider ovarian PRP as ready for prime time as "first line" therapy, it could someday offer another good option for women. And of course this would not just be as a prelude to IVF as initially used, but for general management of menopausal symptoms.

So while ovarian PRP injection has achieved significantly improved AMH and there have been babies born from poor prognosis IVF patients using their own oocytes, the neurobehavioral and metabolic changes could be even more pathbreaking.

If such results can be validated, it would change everything for womankind. Ovarian PRP is positioned to have a reach far beyond any fertility clinic.

"When you arise in the morning,
consider what a precious privilege it is to be alive;
to breathe, to think, to enjoy, to love."

—Marcus Aurelius (121-180)

Rendezvous with Renewal ("The Big Day")

DEAR DIARY—*We arrived in California the day before my PRP appointment on purpose, since everyone knows traffic can be awful. This way we got a good night's rest, woke up early, had a light breakfast and drove over to the clinic to make my 9:30 a.m. appointment. So glad we didn't have to worry about all the airport stress that day!*

After checking in at the clinic, a nurse took me back. There, I sat down in a little chair for a blood draw. I think she took three tubes worth from my arm, although the tourniquet was off before I really knew what happened. I absolutely hate getting my blood drawn, but the equipment she used (a "butterfly" needle) was so tiny I hardly felt anything.

They said it would take about an hour to process the blood sample, so we were given the option to go for coffee or stay put and talk with the doctor while my PRP was getting ready. Since we already had breakfast, I decided to remain at the clinic and meet Dr. Sills in person.

Why not? Over a month before my appointment, I had talked with him (Dr. Sills) by phone. Since then, I had a few other questions. Plus, I just wanted to meet the PRP man before the actual procedure!

That was the right decision. My partner and I were taken into the consult room where Dr. Sills was at his desk. He introduced himself and was very open to address any questions we had, especially issues dealing with "next steps". I took out my list of questions and he said he liked me being so organized and prepared.

All my questions were answered and I found Dr. Sills to be very approachable and eager to help. He fully explained the process that was about to happen.

Dr. Sills even shared some very new research results which, at that time, had not even been published in any medical journal yet. Of all the IVF doctors we have been to, I think he was the one who impressed my partner the most.

Time passed quickly and before long, a nurse knocked on the door to say that my PRP was ready. Dr. Sills again confirmed that I had not recently used any aspirin products. On the way to the procedure room, I stopped briefly at the ladies' room to empty my bladder.

After that little detour I was in the 'PRP room'. I recognized everything. It was the same stuff used for IVF cycle monitoring, something I knew all too well from back home. I put on the paper drape or cover, folded on the end of the exam table for me, and waited for the next step.

Dr. Sills did a brief exam on me; he listened to my heart and lungs with his stethoscope. Then I reclined as if I was getting ready for a Pap test. The ultrasound was carefully placed inside and it reminded me of all those "monitoring scans" I had during my failed IVF cycles last year.

The room lights were dimmed so the ultrasound images could be seen better, and Dr. Sills started measuring things and was calling out the size dimensions of my uterus and ovaries. Someone in the room was writing this all down, and within maybe five minutes it was time for the next step.

I could see Dr. Sills "lining up" one of my ovaries, I think it was my right ovary, on his display screen. Once he was sure everything was safe, I felt a pinch as the needle made its way into that ovary.

He was talking constantly to his nurse, indicating when to start injecting PRP and that nurse was telling him how much of my PRP was going in over time. It was all done in less than a minute!

That was the PRP being injected into my right ovary. The nurse said "We're halfway done, do you want to take a little break?" I told her "No, let's keep going". The level of pain was less than I expected, and it was kind of a relief to feel what it was all about myself. People experience pain differently, but I think the level 2-3 pain (on a one to ten scale) mentioned by the office was about right.

The left ovary was injected next and for this one, I decided to watch the display screen instead of looking up at the ceiling.

I'm glad I did, because I could see my ovary which Dr. Sills had pointed out on the screen, like a little TV set. I was able to watch my PRP material, which appeared white on the monitor, going inside my left ovary. Again, in less than a minute the injection was completed. Now, both ovaries had their PRP.

Dr. Sills then used a speculum to examine my cervix and vagina just to make sure there was no external bleeding. I call that thing "the clamp" and just like at my regular GYN exams, I hate that instrument. But there was no bleeding so the device was out before I could even say anything.

I rested for about 15 minutes, then I got up and got dressed to leave the procedure room. I saw Dr. Sills briefly afterward and he asked how I was feeling, which was a little crampy. Like a period cramp. Just as predicted, by the time we were back in the car everything was normal, with no cramping.

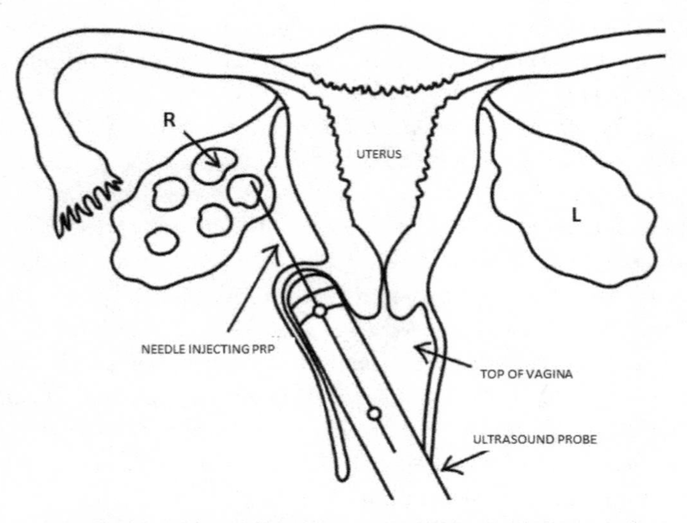

Ovarian Reboot—how it's done. Injection of platelet-derived growth factors into right and left ovaries (R & L) is shown above. Placement of PRP to target is by needle insertion of the activated substrate under trans-vaginal ultrasound guidance. This has been done successfully as an office procedure without anesthesia, taking less than 15 minutes.

As Dr. Sills explained it, what we did was basically like an IVF egg retrieval, except in reverse. With the ovarian PRP procedure, the same kind of equipment is used to put something into ovarian tissue, not to take eggs out, as with IVF egg collection. All in all, it went quickly and I cannot wait to see what happens next with my AMH levels!

My original AMH before the procedure was "undetectable". It was so low that it was off the scale, <0.03. When I got back home, follow-up blood tests were done each month. Dr. Sills said I could get this test every two weeks if I wanted to, and I would have done that, but it just wasn't easy getting to my local lab. I was sure to use the same commercial lab that I used for my testing before the PRP (baseline labs).

The first month after ovarian PRP, I could feel there was something weirdly different in a good way about me, but the AMH blood test showed nothing. The result was still <0.03. So, no change.

Three months later, my AMH had risen to 0.3.

Dr. Sills' office contacted me to set up a phone consult to review everything, and he focused most of his attention bragging on my ovaries and saying how this "ten-fold increase" was a big deal! The reason that surprised me was that my local IVF clinic had consistently refused to work with me if my AMH level was under 1.0, unless egg donor was an option.

By the time three months had passed after my PRP treatment, I was starting to feel much better as a female since a lot of "woman issues" were improving for me. Dr. Sills said that if no IVF clinic in my area would work with me, that his clinic would help.

At this point, my partner and I will be going with his option. At least we know Dr. Sills is familiar with my case, and plus we like him. He asked that we get copies of the "stim sheets" from my prior IVF cycles, and that's what we're waiting on now.

Next stop, IVF ... Wish us luck!

Ovarian Reboot—Frequently Asked Questions

1. Who is the ideal patient for this procedure?

Two options currently exist for ovarian rejuvenation. One is Platelet Rich Plasma (PRP), and a related procedure (enriched platelet factors) increases the level of growth factors derived from platelets. Both involve injecting the patients own cells into her ovarian tissue in an office procedure.

Studies on ovarian response after PRP are only now beginning to appear in medical journals, and there is only one report on healthy pregnancy with IVF following enriched platelet factors.

The only way to determine which treatment best matches a patient's situation is by ongoing research. Accordingly, PRP or enriched platelet factors should be selected by a physician familiar with these two processes on a case by case basis, after reviewing the medical history for each patient.

2. What preliminary data exist on how to select PRP or enriched platelet factors?

The good news is that even if only one ovary can be injected with platelet derived growth factors, this does not appear to diminish the improvement in ovarian reserve. While it is likely that the much higher concentrations of growth signals with enriched platelet factors could yield a superior response, this remains to be conclusively proven.

As presented here, recent work has found that age, weight, and AMH level were not predictive of response after growth factor injection into ovarian tissue. However, baseline platelet count was different. Women with higher platelet levels were more likely to show significant improvements in ovarian reserve. This is why blood tests are recommended before your consult here, so that this information can help guide the decision on which pathway may be best in each situation.

3. Besides fertility enhancement, what other benefits could be expected after this treatment?

This is a key question, because not every patient wants an "ovarian reboot" for IVF or pregnancy. In 2018, a secondary study (via confidential, anonymous questionnaire) was completed based on data from 80 women. The goal of this research was to find out more about 'quality of life' changes they experienced after ovarian PRP. In brief, we learned that even when making new eggs is not the goal, important improvements are still possible for many women.

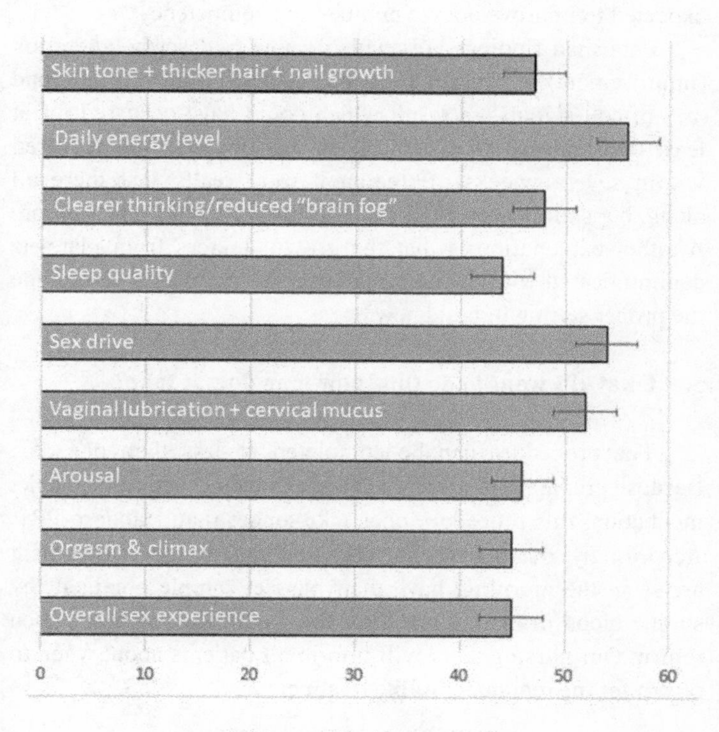

Before vs. After Ovarian PRP
% Improvement

4. How is 'rejuvenation' of the ovaries thought to work?

The treatment involves careful insertion of cytokines, chemokines, and other growth factors into ovarian tissue. These can be thought of as molecular signals which activate cell growth, angiogenesis, and improved blood flow. These changes are expected to improve oocyte number and competency.

Published findings are available now to describe alteration (improvement) in ovarian function after insertion of this broad mix of cell signals—a result which could have occurred for at least two reasons. One scenario is that oocytes we recovered within several weeks of treatment were really just there all along, but simply awakened from dormancy by our intervention. Another explanation is that the growth factors from platelets communicated with uncommitted ovarian stem cells, to provide the proper setting to build new eggs.

5. Okay if I want to do this, how long does it take?

The procedure can be completed in less than one day. Because preparation of enriched platelet factors requires platelet incubation, this procedure does take longer than standard PRP. Accordingly, our patients for enriched platelet factor treatment arrive in the morning, have their platelet sample obtained (by simple blood draw), go out for a few hours for lunch and then return. Our nursing team will inform all patients about when to return for the remainder of the treatment.

6. For 'ovarian rejuvenation' do I need to be on a certain day of my cycle?

No. In the registered clinical trial for ovarian PRP in over 180 women here, many patients were already menopausal so they had no 'cycle day'. Interestingly, some women started having periods again after treatment—a very good sign.

7. Is there any special preparation required before ovarian rejuvenation?

The only medical advice to follow is to get baseline lab tests before you arrive, and more importantly, to avoid aspirin compounds at least two weeks before your appointment. This applies to PRP and enriched platelet factor patients alike, because both treatments depend on platelet health and aspirin is known to have a damaging effect on platelets.

8. What can I expect after treatment...will I feel any different?

The ovarian injection procedures here are very well tolerated. Some patients go back to the airport later the same evening as their procedure here, and there has not been any problem with such travel. On a pain scale of 1 to 10, most patients say this is low, about 2 or 3. This relatively low level of discomfort is why anesthesia is not necessary, as this would have extra risks of its own. Hopefully, after 'ovarian rejuvenation' there will be an improvement across any number of 'female' issues like cervical mucus production, energy level, scalp hair growth, and of course, egg production.

9. How effective is 'ovarian rejuvenation'?

When PRP was evaluated during the registered clinical trial, significant increases in serum AMH (a reliable marker of ovarian reserve) was observed in around 30% of patients. AMH was chosen as the main benchmark because this is the blood test commonly used as a gatekeeper to permit IVF. Some women showed a tenfold post-treatment gain in AMH. We do not yet have data on response following treatment with enriched platelet factors but it is likely to be comparable.

10. If I'm lucky enough to see a response after treatment, how long will I need to wait to see results and how long will it last?

I strongly recommend at least monthly blood testing for AMH to see when a beneficial response happens. Such blood tests can be done anywhere, but for consistency monitoring labs will be done at the same place as baseline (pre-treatment) testing. In general, it takes about three months to see an AMH uptick although some women have shown changes as soon as a few weeks after injection. For fertility patients, IVF should be booked as soon as a sustained increase in AMH is confirmed (usually 90 days later).

Duration of effect is not currently known, only because we do not have extensive longitudinal data to follow-up patients over many years.

However, it seems unlikely that ovarian 'rescue' will be permanent. Some patients have returned for a "booster shot" every 4-6 months, because they find the changes positive and do not want to revert back to the lower pre-treatment level of ovary action.

"The world was to me a secret
which I desired to divine."

—Mary Wollstonecraft Shelley (1797-1851)

Epilogue

Reading this book can pull dreams, almost forgotten, off dusty shelves. Discoveries which at first may appear unrelated, sometimes wait patiently to be bound together.

Stitching those disparate chapters under one cover is not easy. And recent research leads us to this bright library of life, where we read thankfully from atop the shoulders of giants. With sincere hopefulness, we aspire to make a useful contribution to human happiness.

When it comes to recognizing strengths and limits of the adult human ovary, much work remains to be done—here and elsewhere.

What were once thought as the unstoppable and vexing consequences of advancing female age may have, at last, met their match.

From my very first passages here, you saw how one's own battle against the corrosions of low fertility and menopause is but a tiny tile within a much larger mosaic. Yet I admit, the awesome majesty of the creation does nothing to assuage the hurt that any perceived personal failure might render.

My goal here is to place the ovary as the central star in a constellation growing fainter over time. Does misery love company? If yes, then the dimming emptiness of impaired reproduction and failed pregnancy is shared by countless women worldwide.

We have seen not just how genetics direct the ovary to confer female features, but how these same signals drive early egg precursors—we can call them either VSELs or PGCs. To patients, these abbreviations seem like distractions, but the power of these cells is truly impressive.

And there is general agreement now that such "pluripotent" cells which can do anything, they do exist in the adult ovary.

Just having these cells parked someplace in the ovary can't help anyone if they cannot be used. What you have learned here is that growth factors released from platelets, when placed inside sleepy ovaries, can wake them up and "rejuvenate" them out of a state of dormancy.

Finding a way to stimulate older ovaries can't happen unless there is some small population of stem cells available to get the signal.

There's evidence now to verify that such cells are indeed located in older ovaries. This book traces their early beginnings and, more importantly, shows how to coax those cells into action. Because you and your doctor can make this happen using your own platelets, don't expect any multibillion dollar corporations to promote it. In fact, for manufacturers of synthetic hormone products it's really best if the data you now hold in your hand remains obscure.

The language calling for any potential eggs to come forward starts with platelets, acting much like envelopes carrying messages of growth. The information in such letters is powerful, organic, and natural. You are your own postmaster. Without delivering that stimulus package, the older ovary remains in decline and the needle never moves up on the dial to estimate fertility reserve (AMH).

Getting older ovaries in gear to lift their capacity to function has already been described from fertility clinics, first in Greece and also here in California. Most of the women experiencing this after ovarian PRP quickly jump on the AMH wave while its still high, to obtain something other doctors had told them was impossible—their own eggs.

Once you can build that, getting a good embryo and making a baby becomes within your grasp. The number of patients achieving all this is growing, as experience with platelet-derived growth factors becomes better known both in Europe, USA, and beyond.

And yes, there are plenty of woman who don't care about pregnancy. They are simply tired of feeling tired, the brain fog, the cloudy thinking, scalp hair loss, brittle nails & thin skin, vaginal dryness and reduced libido—all features of the transition to menopause.

This list simply reflects hormonal changes thanks to impaired ovaries, as discussed here. We have provided fresh evidence that ovarian PRP delivers growth factors which don't just arrest this crash...it can also rewind its effects. This is an unexpected, unattractive option for anyone hoping to hold every menopausal woman hostage to the synthetic hormone industry.

There's nothing wrong with standard HRT (hormone replacement therapy) when current professional guidelines are followed. Many women have benefitted from HRT. But the work presented here puts a fresh alternative within reach. Is ovarian PRP effective for everyone? Is it a permanent fix? Our research says no, to both questions. But the deck isn't necessarily stacked against ovarian PRP, because standard HRT also gives negative answers to both queries, too.

Familiarity with PRP and its associated growth factors is gaining in acceptance and familiarity from its use in sports medicine, oral surgery, dermatology, and other fields. It now looks like using PRP in reproductive medicine is a strong strategy as well.

Yes. At last, what were once thought as the unstoppable and vexing consequences of advancing female age may have met their match.

We get true progress in clinical medicine from incremental gains, sometimes from unexpected places. The information shared here on ovarian PRP gives a leg up on how this technique may help women attain their personal goals—and a proper reboot can make the first step forward possible.

Best wishes on your personal journey to replenishment and renewal!

Reading List

Abban G, Johnson J (2009). Stem cell support of oogenesis in the human. Hum Reprod 24(12):2974-8.

Atwood CS, Bowen RL (2011). The reproductive-cell cycle theory of aging: an update. Exp Gerontol 46(2-3):100-7.

Bendel-Stenzel M, Anderson R, Heasman J, Wylie C (1998). The origin and migration of primordial germ cells in the mouse. Semin Cell Dev Biol 9(4):393-400.

Betts T, Dutton N, Yarrow H (2001). Epilepsy and the ovary (cutting out the hysteria). Seizure. 10(3):220-8.

Bhartiya D, Anand S, Patel H, Parte S (2017). Making gametes from alternate sources of stem cells: past, present and future. Reprod Biol Endocrinol 15(1):89.

Bhartiya D, Unni S, Parte S, Anand S (2013). Very small embryonic-like stem cells: implications in reproductive biology. Biomed Res Int 2013:682326.

Bowen RL, Atwood CS (2004). Living and dying for sex – a theory of aging based on the modulation of cell cycle signaling by reproductive hormones. Gerontology 50(5):265-90.

Burkart JM, van Schaik C, Griesser M (2017). Looking for unity in diversity: human cooperative childcare in comparative perspective. Proc Biol Sci 284(1869) pii: 20171184.

Byskov AG, Høyer PE, Yding Andersen C *et al* (2011). No evidence for the presence of oogonia in the human ovary after their final clearance during the first two years of life. Hum Reprod 26(8):2129-39.

Castrillon DH, Quade BJ, Wang TY, Quigley C, Crum CP (2000). The human VASA gene is specifically expressed in the germ cell lineage. Proc Natl Acad Sci USA 97(17):9585-90.

Cummins PL, Sills ES, Marron KJ, Harrity C, Walsh DJ, Walsh APH (2016). Impact of Pre-Mixing AMH Serum Samples with Standard Assay Buffer: Ovarian Reserve Estimations and Implications for Clinical IVF Providers. J Reprod Endocrinol Infert 1:10.

De Felici M (2010). Germ stem cells in the mammalian adult ovary: considerations by a fan of the primordial germ cells. Mol Hum Reprod 16(9):632-6.

Eggan K, Jurga S, Gosden R, Min IM, Wagers AJ (2006). Ovulated oocytes in adult mice derive from non-circulating germ cells. Nature 441(7097):1109-14.

Ellis S, Franks DW, Nattrass S *et al* (2018). Postreproductive lifespans are rare in mammals. Ecol Evol 8(5):2482-94.

Greening J (2017). Menopause transition: effects on women's economic participation. HM Government Equalities Office [United Kingdom]; July 20: https://www.gov.uk/government/publications/menopause-transition-effects-on-womenseconomic-participation [site accessed May 15, 2019].

Guigon CJ, Cohen-Tannoudji M (2011). Reconsidering the roles of female germ cells in ovarian development and folliculogenesis. Biol Aujourdhui 205(4):223-33.

Havens AM, Shiozawa Y, Jung Y *et al* (2013). Human very small embryonic-like cells generate skeletal structures, in vivo. Stem Cells Dev 22(4):622-30.

Hawkes K, O'Connell JF, Jones NG, Alvarez H, Charnov EL (1998). Grandmothering, menopause, and the evolution of human life histories. Proc Natl Acad Sci USA 95(3):1336-9.

Hosseini L, Shirazi A, Naderi MM *et al* (2017). Platelet-rich plasma promotes the development of isolated human primordial and primary follicles to the preantral stage. Reprod Biomed Online 35(4):343-350.

Hsueh AJ, Kawamura K, Cheng Y, Fauser BC (2015). Intraovarian control of early folliculogenesis. Endocr Rev 36(1):1-24.

Hummitzsch K, Anderson RA, Wilhelm D *et al* (2015). Stem cells, progenitor cells, and lineage decisions in the ovary. Endocr Rev 36(1):65-91.

Imudia AN, Wang N, Tanaka Y, White YA, Woods DC, Tilly JL (2013). Comparative gene expression profiling of adult mouse ovary-derived oogonial stem cells supports a distinct cellular identity. Fertil Steril 100(5):1451-8.

Jing Y, Li L, Li YY *et al* (2019). Embryo quality, and not chromosome nondiploidy, affects mitochondrial DNA content in mouse blastocysts. J Cell Physiol 234(7):10481-8.

Johnson J, Canning J, Kaneko T, Pru JK, Tilly JL (2004). Germline stem cells and follicular renewal in the postnatal mammalian ovary. Nature 428(6979):145-50.

Kucia M, Maj M, Mierzejewska K, Shin DM, Ratajczak J, Ratajczak MZ (2013). Challenging dogmas - or how much evidence is necessary to claim that there is a direct developmental and functional link between the primordial germ cell (PGC) lineage and hematopoiesis? [Abstract 1215] 55th ASH Annual Meeting Blood 2013; 122:21.

Lacci KM, Dardik A (2010). Platelet-rich plasma: support for its use in wound healing. Yale J Biol Med 83(1):1-9.

Le Bouffant R, Souquet B, Duval N *et al* (2011). Msx1 and Msx2 promote meiosis initiation. Development 138(24):5393-402.

Lee HJ, Selesniemi K, Niikura Y *et al* (2007). Bone marrow transplantation generates immature oocytes and rescues long-term fertility in a preclinical mouse model of chemotherapy-induced premature ovarian failure. J Clin Oncol 25(22):3198-204.

Levitis DA, Burger O, Lackey LB (2013). The human post-fertile lifespan in comparative evolutionary context. Evol Anthropol 22(2):66-79.

Loewenberg S (2009). James Vaupel: an innovator in the demography of ageing. Lancet 374:1139.

Lütje W (2005). Menstruation in the systemic context. New questions—questionable connections. Zentralbl Gynakol 127(5):329-32.

Marie-Scemama L, Even M, De La Joliniere JB, Ayoubi JM (2019). Endometriosis and the menopause: why the question merits our full attention. Horm Mol Biol Clin Investig 37(2) DOI: 10.1515/hmbci-2018-0071.

Møllgård K, Jespersen A, Lutterodt MC, Yding Andersen C, Høyer PE, Byskov AG (2010). Human primordial germ cells migrate along nerve fibers and Schwann cells from the dorsal hind gut mesentery to the gonadal ridge. Mol Hum Reprod 16(9):621-31.

Morrison C (2019). US fertility falls to record low, fewest births in 32 years. Washington Examiner [*newspaper*];May 15:A4.

Nurden AT (2011). Platelets, inflammation and tissue regeneration. Thromb Haemost 105 Suppl 1:S13-33.

Pantos K, Nitsos N, Kokkali G *et al* (2016). Ovarian rejuvenation and folliculogenesis reactivation in peri-menopausal women after autologous platelet-rich plasma treatment. In: Abstracts, ESHRE 32nd Annual Meeting [Helsinki] 3-6 July. Hum Reprod 2016 (Suppl1):i301.

Park ES, Woods DC, Tilly JL (2013). Bone morphogenetic protein 4 promotes mammalian oogonial stem cell differentiation via Smad1/5/8 signaling. Fertil Steril 100(5):1468-75.

Parte S, Bhartiya D, Telang J *et al* (2011). Detection, characterization, and spontaneous differentiation in vitro of very small embryonic-like putative stem cells in adult mammalian ovary. Stem Cells Dev 20(8):1451-64.

Powledge TM (2008). Origin of menopause: Why do women outlive fertility? Sci Am; April 3. https://www.scientificamerican.com/article/the-origin-of-menopause/ [site accessed May 15, 2019].

Ratajczak MZ, Zuba-Surma E, Wojakowski W *et al* (2014). Very small embryonic-like stem cells (VSELs) represent a real challenge in stem cell biology: recent pros and cons in the midst of a lively debate. Leukemia 28(3):473-84.

Reizel Y, Itzkovitz S, Adar R *et al* (2012). Cell lineage analysis of the mammalian female germline. PLoS Genet 8(2):e1002477.

Robin C, Ottersbach K, de Bruijn M, Ma X, van der Horn K, Dzierzak E (2003). Developmental origins of hematopoietic stem cells. Oncol Res 13(6-10):315-21.

Šaffa G, Kubicka AM, Hromada M, Kramer KL (2019). Is the timing of menarche correlated with mortality and fertility rates? PLoS One 14(4):e0215462.

Sfakianoudis K, Simopoulou M, Nitsos N *et al* (2018). A Case Series on Platelet-Rich Plasma Revolutionary Management of Poor Responder Patients. Gynecol Obstet Invest 1-8 doi: 10.1159/000491697.

Shin DM, Zuba-Surma EK, Wu W *et al* (2009). Novel epigenetic mechanisms that control pluripotency and quiescence of adult bone marrow-derived Oct4(+) very small embryonic-like stem cells. Leukemia 23(11):2042-51.

Sills ES, Kirman I, Thatcher SS 3rd, Palermo GD (1998). Sex-selection of human spermatozoa: evolution of current techniques and applications. Arch Gynecol Obstet 261(3):109-15.

Sills ES, Sholes TE, Perloe M, Kaplan CR, Davis JG, Tucker MJ (2002). Characterization of a novel receptor mutation A-->T at exon 4 in complete androgen insensitivity syndrome and a carrier sibling via bidirectional polymorphism sequence analysis. Int J Mol Med 9(1):45-8.

Sills ES, Takeuchi T, Tucker MJ, Palermo GD (2004). Genetic and epigenetic modifications associated with human ooplasm donation and mitochondrial heteroplasmy—considerations for interpreting studies of heritability and reproductive outcome. Med Hypotheses 62(4):612-7.

Sills ES, Alper MM, Walsh AP (2009). Ovarian reserve screening in infertility: practical applications and theoretical directions for research. Eur J Obstet Gynecol Reprod Biol 146(1):30-6.

Sills ES, Palermo GD (2013). Gonadotropin releasing hormone in the primitive vertebrate family Myxinidae: reproductive neuroanatomy and evolutionary aspects. Neuroendocrinol Lett 34(3):177-83.

Sills ES (2013). An evidence-based policy for the provision of subsidised fertility treatment in California: Integration of array comparative genomic hybridisation with IVF and mandatory single embryo transfer to lower multiple gestation and preterm birth rates [PhD thesis]. Univ Westminster (Lond); EtHOS British Library Record: https://ethos.bl.uk/OrderDetails.do?uin=uk.bl.ethos.576982

Sills ES, Rickers NS, Li X, Palermo GD (2018). First data on in vitro fertilization and blastocyst formation after intraovarian injection of calcium gluconate-activated autologous platelet rich plasma. Gynecol Endocrinol 34(9):756-760.

Sills ES, Li X, Rickers NS, Petersen JL, Rickers JM, Wood SH (2019). Intraovarian injection of autologous platelet rich plasma: longitudinal data on ovarian reserve patterns measured in 182 poor-prognosis IVF patients. J Obstet Gynaecol 2019: *in press.*

Sills ES, Rickers NS, Svid S, Rickers JM, Wood SH (2019). Normalized ploidy following 20 consecutive blastocysts with chromosomal error: healthy 46,XY pregnancy with IVF after intraovarian injection of autologous enriched platelet-derived growth factors. Int J Mol Cell Med 2019: *in press.*

Sills ES, Li X, Rickers NS, Wood SH, Palermo GD (2019). Metabolic and neurobehavioral response following intraovarian administration of autologous activated platelet rich plasma: First qualitative data. Neuroendocrinol Lett 39(6):427-433.

Sills ES, Wood SH (2019). Autologous activated platelet rich plasma injection into adult human ovary tissue: Molecular mechanism, analysis, and discussion of reproductive response. Biosci Rep May 15. pii: BSR20190805.

Stein G (2010). Hannah: a case of infertility and depression—psychiatry in the Old Testament. Br J Psychiatry 197(6):492.

Stévant I, Papaioannou MD, Nef S (2018). A brief history of sex determination. Mol Cell Endocrinol 468:3-10.

Szafarowska M, Jerzak M (2013). Ovarian aging and infertility. Ginekol Pol 84(4):298-304.

Tsiligiannis S, Panay N, Stevenson JC (2019). Premature ovarian insufficiency and long-term health consequences. Curr Vasc Pharmacol Jan 21. doi: 10.2174/1570161117666190122101611.

Virant-Klun I, Zech N, Rozman P *et al* (2008). Putative stem cells with an embryonic character isolated from the ovarian surface epithelium of women with no naturally present follicles and oocytes. Differentiation 76(8):843-56.

Wang H, Jiang M, Bi H, Chen X, He L, Li X, Wu J (2014). Conversion of female germline stem cells from neonatal and prepubertal mice into pluripotent stem cells. J Mol Cell Biol 6(2):164-71.

White YA, Woods DC, Takai Y, Ishihara O, Seki H, Tilly JL (2012). Oocyte formation by mitotically active germ cells purified from ovaries of reproductive-age women. Nat Med 18(3):413-21.

Willekens, FJ (2014). Demographic transitions in Europe and the world. Max Planck Institute for Demographic Research (Working Paper) WP-2014-004:1-32.

Xie W, Wang H, Wu J (2014). Similar morphological and molecular signatures shared by female and male germline stem cells. Sci Rep 4:5580.

Zhang Y, Wu J (2009). Molecular cloning and characterization of a new gene, Oocyte-G1. J Cell Physiol 218(1):75-83.

Zhang Y, Yang Z, Yang Y *et al* (2011). Production of transgenic mice by random recombination of targeted genes in female germline stem cells. J Mol Cell Biol 3(2):132-41.

Zou K, Hou L, Sun K, Xie W, Wu J (2011). Improved efficiency of female germline stem cell purification using fragilis-based magnetic bead sorting. Stem Cells Dev 20(12):2197-204.

Zou K, Yuan Z, Yang Z *et al* (2009). Production of offspring from a germline stem cell line derived from neonatal ovaries. Nat Cell Biol 11(5):631-6.

Zuckerman S (1952). The number of oocytes in the mature ovary. Rec Prog Horm Res 6:63–109.

Appendix

Bioscience Reports (2019) **39** BSR20190805
https://doi.org/10.1042/BSR20190805

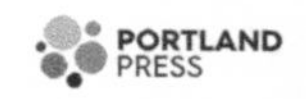

Hypothesis

Autologous activated platelet-rich plasma injection into adult human ovary tissue: molecular mechanism, analysis, and discussion of reproductive response

E. Scott Sills[1,2] and Samuel H. Wood[1]

[1]Gen 5 Fertility Center, Office for Reproductive Research, Center for Advanced Genetics; San Diego, CA, U.S.A.; [2]Applied Biotechnology Research Group, University of Westminster; London W1B 2HW, U.K.

Correspondence: E. Scott Sills (drsills@CAGivf.com)

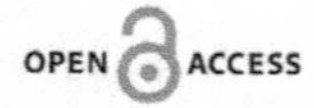

In clinical infertility practice, one intractable problem is low (or absent) ovarian reserve which in turn reflects the natural oocyte depletion associated with advancing maternal age. The number of available eggs has been generally thought to be finite and strictly limited, an entrenched and largely unchallenged tenet dating back more than 50 years. In the past decade, it has been suggested that renewable ovarian germline stem cells (GSCs) exist in adults, and that such cells may be utilized as an oocyte source for women seeking to extend fertility. Currently, the issue of whether mammalian females possess such a population of renewable GSCs remains unsettled. The topic is complex and even agreement on a definitive approach to verify the process of 'ovarian rescue' or 're-potentiation' has been elusive. Similarities have been noted between wound healing and ovarian tissue repair following capsule rupture at ovulation. In addition, molecular signaling events which might be necessary to reverse the effects of reproductive ageing seem congruent with changes occurring in tissue injury responses elsewhere. Recently, clinical experience with such a technique based on autologous activated platelet-rich plasma (PRP) treatment of the adult human ovary has been reported. This review summarizes the present state of understanding of the interaction of platelet-derived growth factors with adult ovarian tissue, and the outcome of human reproductive potential following PRP treatment.

Received: 29 March 2019
Revised: 09 May 2019
Accepted: 14 May 2019

Accepted Manuscript Online: 15 May 2019
Version of Record published: 04 June 2019

Background

An important aspect of successful IVF is the surgical recovery of an adequate number of oocytes for prompt and monitored fertilization (usually via ICSI). It is the paucity of this essential egg contribution which is typically foreshadowed by laboratory tests indicating diminished reserve [1]. The availability of mature oocytes for IVF is in fact the closing chapter in a long signaling narrative within the ovary, evolving from multiple events. This seems to begin with the development of the ovary itself, reaching a conclusion at the crescendo moment of ovulation. Throughout this journey, the oocyte precursor which acts as a central passenger is accompanied by supporting somatic cells to enable survival and eventual maturation of the egg. For example, the growing germ cells gradually become vested with epithelial elements known as 'ovigerous cords' comprising pregranulosa cells. As ovarian development concludes, these ovigerous cords splinter off into individual primordial follicles—consisting of the oocyte surrounded by its companion single layer of granulosa cells.

Bioscience Reports (2019) **39** BSR20190805
https://doi.org/10.1042/BSR20190805

The ovary: its development and actions

Acting primarily to sustain oocyte development and to produce maturational hormones necessary for puberty, the adult ovary is the key regulator of the reproductive cycle and pregnancy over the course of the female reproductive career. These myriad functions require a constant cascade of remodeling and regression, entailing considerable biochemical and tissue reorganization [2]. Of note, several pathological ovarian conditions including polycystic ovary syndrome, premature ovarian insufficiency/failure, and ovarian malignancies have all been linked with disturbances in how cells within the ovary behave. Early work with several novel interventions has suggested ways to improve ovarian response during IVF, but, with uncertainty. In fact, more questions have emerged as findings from pilot studies are assessed. In the meantime, any effort to enhance or extend fertility must be predicated on the fullest possible knowledge of the cell and tissue remodeling processes which occur in the ovary.

An understanding of the developmental origins of the ovary may be guided by observations from comparative anatomy with related structures, particularly testis and adrenal. Yet in the special case of the ovary, there is one characteristic which sets it apart from most other physiologic systems—unlike other female endocrine organs, the ovary undergoes special functional and morphological modifications at puberty. Even during early embryological development, ovarian morphogenesis is far from simple. As mesonephric derivatives, the gonads follow distinct developmental pathways for males and females but do transit a brief phase of bipotentiality before committing to their developmental destiny. Moreover, some ovarian components actually originate outside the organ and arrive later as imports [3]. This would include primordial germ cells (PGCs) (from yolk sac) and certain immune cells (from dorsal aorta); sources for some somatic cell types still remain unclear [4].

This interplay between germ cells and somatic cells appears critical, as fragmentation of ovigerous cords into independent follicles does not occur in the absence of germ cells. Thus proper female differentiation of ovarian somatic cells is modulated by the oocyte itself, as the latter appears to inhibit the testis-differentiating sequence to conserve the fate of adjacent pregranulosa cells (instead of developing into Sertoli cells, for example). In this milieu, primordial follicles continue to be recruited into the growing follicle population to develop through primary, preantral, antral, and preovulatory stages before being released at ovulation. The oocyte also governs the functional differentiation of granulosa cells, preventing their premature maturation into luteal cells in the final stages of growth [5].

Parallel to the tandem, symbiotic relationship between germ cells and somatic cells coordinating their actions to yield follicles, evidence now exists to show that some germ cells are present on or near the ovarian surface [6,7]. With lateral stromal expansion under the ovarian capsule, the once 'open' ovigerous cords eventually close and become isolated from the surface, thus marooning some epithelial cells and some egg precursors at the ovarian surface [8]. What is the developmental purpose of this process, and what evolutionary advantage is conferred by it? While the function of these stranded germ cells is not known, some seem to be lost from the ovarian surface into the periovarian space [9,10] or undergo local atresia. It could be that these are the source of GSCs (germline stem cells) which have been isolated from surface or outer cortex regions of the ovary [11].

Ovarian GSCs: sources and destinations

The reason these cells matter to current fertility practice is that, at least for the past half century, clinicians have worked under the assumption that the entire reserve of oocytes is fixed at birth. Human ovaries are not supposed to have the potential to receive any deposits to this account after this time. Moreover from this oocyte endowment, only withdrawals are possible over a lifetime until the balance is depleted, reaching zero at menopause [12]. This classical ovarian reserve concept met a serious challenge in 2004, and reignited a debate regarding whether oogenesis might be possible in mammals far into adulthood [13]. Specifically, putative GSCs (oogonial stem cells) have been reported to exist in the ovaries of adult humans [11], mice [14], and rats [15]. The first description of renewal of germ cells in postnatal mice ovaries was more than 10 years ago, after examining changes in follicle numbers with age [13]. These investigators subsequently found expression of germline markers in bone marrow-derived cells [16]. Interestingly, bone marrow and peripheral blood transplantations resulted in recovery of oocyte production in wild-type mice sterilized by chemotherapy and ataxia telangiectasia-mutated mice. From this, it was concluded that bone marrow and peripheral blood might be a potential source of female germ cells that could permit egg production in adulthood.

Curiously, a parabiosis experiment [17] failed to support this finding, in which the vasculature of wild-type mice was surgically grafted to that of transgenic mice expressing green fluorescent protein (GFP) under the control of the β-actin promoter. Even though high levels of blood cell chimerism were noted, no GFP-positive germ cells were ovulated in the non-transgenic mice [17]. Further research focused on effects of bone marrow transplantation from TgOG2 transgenic mice with germline-specific expression of GFP (Oct4-GFP) into recipients depleted of ovarian follicles due to cyclophosphamide and busulfan exposure [18]. Bone marrow-derived germ cells have been found

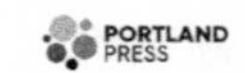

in primordial and immature growing follicles, but these did not advance to the ovulatory stage. It was also shown that bone marrow-derived germ cells were not CD45^{+} monocytes, and Oct4-GFP is not exclusively specific to germ cells, as this marker is also expressed in other adult stem cell populations and tumors [17,19]. Thus, the possibility exists that GFP+ cells noted in recipient mice were actually macrophages [18] since they lacked the typical morphology of oocytes and Oct4+ macrophages seen previously in rabbit tissue in association with atherosclerotic plaque [20]. Such apparently conflicting findings could be explained by considering that transplanted bone marrow-derived (or blood-borne leukocytes) do not actually replace ovarian germ cells, but rather support their development and recovery from radio- or chemotherapy [19].

It is now recognized that the immune system plays an important supportive role in ovarian function, particularly with respect to follicle development [21,22]. Recent work has found a population of CD4^{+}CD25^{+}FOXP3^{+} Treg cells to be especially relevant, and these cells from females exhibit a more potent suppressive function than similar cells obtained from males [23]. Interestingly, this sex-specific effect can be reversed if males are grafted with ovarian tissue [24], demonstrating an antigen-specific Treg suppression and the need for sustained presence of the cognate tissue antigen to produce ovary antigen-specific Treg cells. Dysfunction of normal immunomodulatory function in the ovary—particularly loss of Treg cells—has been suggested as a cause for premature ovarian insufficiency in some cases [25].

So where do eggs ultimately come from? It seems unlikely that oocytes arise from a hematopoietic stem cell source. This mechanism was refuted by data from a study using a 'molecular clock' method to estimate the number of cellular mitotic divisions since arising from zygote stage [26]. The approach followed specific (somatic) mutations to develop lineage trees, predicated on the concept that spontaneous mutations in DNA can be used to count the number of mitotic divisions ('depth') a cell has undergone since soon after fertilization; in this way mutation patterns in multiple loci can reveal the lineage relations among individual cells. Thus an assembly-line model of oocyte activation was advanced, whereby the earliest oocytes eligible for ovulation are also those which enter meiosis first [27]. Importantly, the 'mitotic age' or 'depth' of oocytes was found to be different across mesenchymal and hematopoietic stem cells of bone marrow origin [26], making it difficult to show that oocytes are seeded from bone marrow cells.

Almost 10 years ago, a key development was reported when a population of mitotically active cells discovered in immature and adult mouse ovaries were successfully manipulated *in vitro* to evoke germline characteristics [14]. The isolation of such cells, however, was insufficient to prove definitively that they are involved in postnatal oogenesis. Indeed, the ovary-derived cells were different from bone marrow-derived cells, exhibiting stable expression of germline markers such as Oct4, MVH, Dazl, Blimp1, Fragilis, Stella, and Rex1 [14]. Using a transplantation model to repopulate cells in murine ovaries affected by chemotherapy exposure, it was shown that these cells might be ovarian GSCs. Moreover, *de novo* oocytes were identified and were capable of fertilization, resulting in birth of live offspring carrying a traceable genetic marker introduced into the cells before transplantation. Mating of this generation with wild-type mice produced transgenic offspring, which inherited the marker via transgene germline transmission [14]. To explain this, it has been theorized that the ovary capsule (epithelium) might be the source of GSCs, because immunohistochemical studies have found cells double-positive for both mouse vasa homolog (MVH) and the proliferation marker 5-bromodeoxyuridine [13,14]. Using a female transgenic mouse model expressing GFP regulated by Oct4 promoter, a GFP-positive cell population was found near ovary epithelium in adult mice [28]. Such GFP-positive cells were stable in culture for up to 1 year and expressed several germ cell-specific markers (GCNA [germ cell nuclear antigen], cKIT, MVH) with sustained telomerase activity. The culture of these GSCs with granulosa cells of neonatal mice did enable development of follicle-like structures, but their functionality remains untested.

Cultured GSCs expressing GFP from neonatal and adult mice have been transferred into chemotherapy-pretreated recipient mice, producing transgenic F1 and F2 offspring [29]. Transfection of GSCs with recombinant viruses carrying Oocyte-G1, Dnaic2 (mouse dynein axonemal intermediate chain 2) or liposome-mediated transfection with an Oocyte-G1 knockdown vector, yielded heterozygous offspring after transplantation into chemotherapy-pretreated mice. No transgenic offspring were observed after transplantation of short-term cultured and GFP-transfected oocytes, providing evidence that the transgenic offspring following transplantation of GFP-positive GSCs were not from oocytes [29,30]. Comparisons of gene expression profiles among embryonic stem cells, PGCs, GSCs (fresh isolates), and cultured GSCs from adult mice revealed that the profile of PGCs was highly concordant with embryonic stem cells, whereas fresh GSCls did not express the pluripotency-associated genes *Zfp296* (encoding zinc finger protein 296), *Utf1* (undifferentiated embryonic cell transcript factor-1), *Nanog*, and *Sox2* (SRY box 2) [31]. Cultured GSCs did resemble PGC markers however, as Zfp296, Utf1, Nanog, and Sox2 all were present. Interestingly, these cultured GSCs also weakly expressed Stra8 (stimulated by retinoic acid 8), a marker of cell entry into meiosis.

The efficiency of conversion for such cells into oocytes appears very low [32]. While it may be that less than 1% of seeded GSCs spontaneously differentiate into oocyte-like cells expressing Stra8, this oocyte conversion yield was doubled with the addition of BMP4 (bone morphogenetic protein 4), known to assist induction of PGCs in mouse embryos [33]. These oocyte-like cells demonstrated much higher Stra8, Msx1 (muscle segment homeobox 1) and Msx2 expression [32], regarded as BMP-responsive genes in human and mouse fetal ovaries [34,35].

Given the importance of these findings it was not entirely surprising that other researchers critiqued the nature and consistency of cells isolated, as well as the laboratory protocol used to produce them [36]. An improved fluorescence methodology was later suggested to isolate and purify GSCs [11], in support of earlier work which concluded primitive germ cells could produce fertilizable oocytes and embryos. GSCs have also been derived from adult human ovaries, cultured *in vitro*, and shown after injection into human ovarian cortex cells to develop into what look like immature oocytes (validated by gene marker labeling); these were later enclosed by granulosa cells to form follicles [11].

It should be noted that there is no agreement on the preferred technique to isolate GSCs. Relying on DDX4/MVH expression to isolate and purify GSCs is problematic since DDX4 (a type of RNA helicase) can also be present in germ cell cytoplasm [37]. Cells isolated without permeabilization have expressed other germline markers like Dppa3, Prdm1, Dazl, Tert (telomerase reverse transcriptase), and Ifitm3 (Fragilis), but not oocyte-specific markers such as Zp3 (zona pellucida sperm binding protein 3), Nobox (newborn ovary homeobox protein), or Gdf9 (growth differentiation factor 9). This suggests the existence of 'immature' germline cells in the ovary, capable of expressing DDX4 or domains of DDX4 on the cell surface. DDX4 might become silenced in undifferentiated GSCs by insertion into the cell membrane, and after commitment to the oocyte fate, DDX4 is no longer externally expressed [31]. Other methods to identify and isolate (murine) GSCs with improved efficiency using antibodies and antibody-assisted magnetic-bead sorting have also been reported [38]. In any case, female GSCs obtained from prepubertal or neonatal mice have been induced to become pluripotent embryonic stem-like cells under specified culture conditions [39] and these GSCs have characteristics similar to male GSCs/spermatogonial stem cells [40].

Pathways to the oocyte

The developmental lineage of human eggs has received considerable investigative attention [41]. Their cellular ancestor (the PGC) is known to appear very early in embryonic life. In mice, precursors of PGCs have been identified as early as embryonic day (E) 6 or 6.5 [42]. Such PGCs precursors develop under the control of signals including BMP2, 4, and 8, and are characterized by expression of PR domain containing 1 (PRDM1 or BLIMP1), PRDM14, and up-regulation of Fragilis (also known as IFITM3 or interferon-induced transmembrane protein 3). Within the first week of embryo development (E7), small clusters of PGCs stabilized by E-cadherin arrive posterior to the primitive streak in the extraembryonic mesoderm. PGCs express TNAP (a non-specific alkaline phosphatase) and DPPA3 (developmental pluripotency associated 3, also known as Stella) at about this time. Soon afterward PGCs migrate to the hindgut and, via dorsal mesentery, into the developing genital ridges. During this migration process, PGCs still express TNAP but also OCT3/4 (octamer-binding transcription factor 3/4; also known as POU5F1), the proto-oncogene cKIT, and SSEA (stage-specific embryonic antigen) 1 and 3. By the time the murine embryo enters its 12th day (E12), most PGCs have already arrived at the genital ridges. Human PGCs are first identified at gestational week 3 (E21) in the dorsal wall of the yolk sac, near the developing allantois [43]. By the time genital ridges develop by week 5, the PGCs have migrated from the hindgut to the dorsal mesentery and then further laterally, to colonize these structures.

There is now general agreement that *in vitro* differentiation of PGCs into gametes is indeed the crucial step and remains a major bottleneck [17]. PGCs are first seen in the proximal epiblast around E7 in mice, migrate via the aorta-gonad-mesonephros region, ultimately settling in the gonadal ridge to proliferate in large number (to approximately 25000 cells) as the second week approaches. There exists an intriguing overlap between PGCs migration along the dorsal mesentery and primitive hematopoiesis which is initiated at about the same time [18]. Being pluripotent, PGCs can produce both germ cells as well as hematopoietic cells. Prior to the second week, genital ridge PGCs stop dividing (female cells enter meiosis; male cells show mitotic arrest). Oogonia are formed in females next, whereas in males these become gonocytes.

At birth, gonocytes undergo rapid proliferation to form spermatogonia which further proliferate and differentiate into spermatocytes, next undergoing meiosis and later forming sperm. Crucially, a small number of spermatogonial stem cells with the ability to self-renew and further differentiate into sperm remain in the testis throughout adult life. A related cell set with small diameter (3–6 μm) is notable for long telomeres and pluripotent markers such as Oct-4, Nanog, Rex-1, SSEA-1 (in mice) and SSEA-4 (in humans); these are termed very small embryonic-like stem cells (VSELs). These pluripotent VSELs have been reported in adult tissues including gonads; they are relatively quiescent, have sufficient resilience to survive radiation and remain present in senescent, non-functional gonads. VSELs can be sorted as Sca^{+} LIN-$CD45^{-}$ in mice and as $CD133^{+}$LIN-$CD45^{-}$ in humans. As with embryonic stem cells, VSELs stain positive for alkaline phosphatase, have a distinct spherical shape with a large nucleus surrounded by a thin

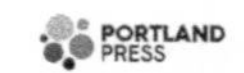

rim of cytoplasm and high nuclear:cytoplasmic ratio. Interestingly, mouse bone marrow VSELs have been shown to have transcriptionally active chromatin elements for both Oct-4 and Nanog promoters [44]. Their pluripotent state is shown by their ability to self-renew and differentiate *in vitro* into all three germ layers in both mice and humans [45,46]. VSELs mobilize in circulation in response to injury to regenerate damaged tissues and also in response to G-CSF treatment [47–49].

Being functionally and developmentally equivalent to PGCs (as natural precursors to gametes), VSELs may spontaneously differentiate into gametes *in vitro*. Niche cells such as Sertoli cells in the male (and mesenchymal cells in the female) can be transplanted and restore gonadal function by providing paracrine support to endogenous VSELs. Such an approach has been used successfully in animal studies and has resulted in a livebirth in a woman with premature ovarian failure [50]. These VSELs are the PGCs which migrate to the gonadal ridge during early embryonic development and persist long after the postnatal period [43].

Such similarities notwithstanding, there are some key contrasts between migrating PGCs (15–20 μm) and VSELs (3–6 μm); additional research is needed to establish whether VSELs are more developmentally primitive than PGCs. It is plausible that PGCs could actually be a precursor to pluripotent stem cells *in vitro*, although they do not seem to behave as stem cells *in vivo*. Indeed, later in fetal development the true stem cell population of SSCs appears in the testis and divides throughout life, yielding ongoing spermatogenesis. The ovary could have comparable cells with stem-like characteristics capable of differentiating into oocytes, yet controversy remains on this point [51,52].

Expression of pluripotency transcription factors is lost after gastrulation in most epiblast stem cells, and these develop further into somatic structures. VSELs present in adult tissues might actually be PGCs, or their precursors [53]. Such a hypothesis is supported from observations that both PGCs and VSELs are pluripotent and relatively quiescent, and this shared quiescence is secondary to similar epigenetic modification of (paternally) imprinted genes including *Igf2-H19* and *KCNK1p57*. In addition, both PGCs and VSELs express Stella, Fragilis, Blimp1, MVH; late migrating markers specific to PGCs such as MVH, Dppa 2, Dppa4, Sall4 are also expressed by VSELs. VSELs also express several miRNAs that dampen Igf-1/Igf-2 signaling in these cells (mir681, mir470, mir669b) as well as up-regulate expression of p57 (mir25.1, mir19b, mir92). Similarities continue in that VSELs have also been found to express functional receptors for genes involved in PGC development into gametes. VSELs found in gonads and bone marrow may explain the observed plasticity and the ability of bone marrow cells to differentiate into germ cells [54]. Given the developmental origin of VSELs, their proliferation, like PGCs, is controlled by DNA methylation status of several imprinted genes (*e.g*., Rasgrf1, H19, and Igf2). During cellular senescence such proliferation-repressive epigenetic factors gradually disappear. This causes an increased sensitivity to Ins/Igf signaling, which in turn leads to depletion of VSELs [55].

Interestingly, a direct developmental link between PGCs and hematopoiesis may also exist [45]. Considerable overlap exists among chromosomal aberrations seen in germline tumors and leukemias/lymphomas, suggesting they share a common clonal origin with precursor VSELs. Thus it could be that a VSEL population exists in adults, undergoing hematopoiesis in bone marrow, and gametogenesis in the gonads. This concept fundamentally challenges accepted thinking that PGCs migrate exclusively to the gonadal ridge to yield germ cells. Rather, migration to various tissues by PGCs may occur, persisting well into adulthood to serve as a reserve pool for tissue committed stem cells [54]. Yet defining, locating, and isolating the cells that fulfil pluripotency criteria remains controversial, underscoring the importance of characterizing the cellular phenotype of these cells more completely [56]. But even when reliable techniques to harvest such cells become available, what will be the next step?

Follicular development, recruitment, and ovulation

Follicles within the ovary may be tracked back (anatomically) to the differentiation of the oogonia within primordial follicles (see Figure 1), although steps essential to activation of primordial follicles (physiologically) may revert even further and are incompletely characterized. What is known is that some follicles join a gradually enlarging primary follicle cohort, thereby beginning a journey which terminates either at ovulation or follicular atresia. Along this developmental course, what switching mechanisms determine the destiny of each member? It appears that this sequence is regulated by intrinsic factors generated by somatic elements of the ovary, especially granulosa and theca cells. Operating in concert, these two compartments produce signals required for the follicle to advance to late preantral or early antral development. The endocrine effects of FSH and LH are needed to sustain further follicular growth; atresia is generally the consequence of the failure to receive or process such gonadotropin signaling. As a follicle approaches its periovulatory phase, other players join the signaling orchestra including prostaglandins, steroids, and proteins of the epidermal growth factor family. While the precise measure and contribution of each signal member require additional study, it is clear that the achievement of follicle maturation entails a sophisticated program of regulatory mediators of both somatic and germ cell origin [57]. Ovarian surface epithelium derives from the mesodermal lining

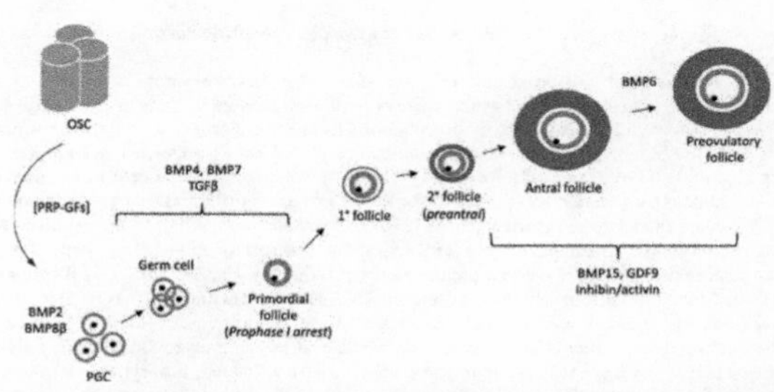

Figure 1. Recruitment and growth of oocytes, from PGC stage through mature follicle, illustrating various growth factors mediating development

Known components of this sequence include granulosa precursors (red), theca compartment (blue), and germ cells (black). Upstream contributions by ovarian stem cells (OSC) may be possible under conditions enabled by growth factors released by platelet-rich plasma (PRP-GFs). Other relevant regulators are BMP2, BMP6, and BMP8β, which are involved in cytokine–cytokine receptor interactions; and Transforming growth factor β (TGF-β), which activates various substrates and regulatory proteins inducing transcription of genes for differentiation, chemotaxis, and proliferation. Later direction is under control of BMP15, a paracrine signal exclusively expressed in ovarian tissue which is involved in oocyte and follicular growth, as well as GDF9, a down-regulator of inhibin-A and promoter of further follicular maturation.

of the intraembryonic coelom and nearby areas where the gonad is formed [58,59]. However, when the bovine fetal ovary first develops it is not at first vested with a defined surface epithelium underlaid by a basal lamina (as observed in the adult), except at the base of the ovary where it arises from the mesonephros [60,61].

It may be that the nascent ovary begins as a cluster of gonadal ridge epithelial like (GREL) cells, which themselves proliferate from the mesonephric surface epithelium, in a process that is also associated with degradation of the basal lamina. This allows the PGCs then to associate with adjacent GREL cells. It has been observed that the mesonephric surface epithelium is single-layered, except where gonadal thickening occurs [62]. The stroma does not penetrate into the ovary until later, and GREL cells on the surface eventually become epithelium only after the stroma has expanded to just underneath the GREL cells [60]. Even though a defined surface epithelium is lacking in the early ovary, the ovarian hilum is an exception where a mesonephric protrusion exists, covered by surface epithelium with a subepithelial basal lamina and epithelial–stromal interface which directly originates from the mesonephros [60]. The rest of the ovary derives its surface epithelial cells from GREL cells. This may be relevant since the surface epithelium of the adult mouse ovary is not uniform, as the base (hilum) of the mouse ovary has stem cells with greater oncogenic potential compared with cells at other ovarian surface locations [61,62]. It is plausible that these differing developmental origins of ovarian epithelial cells (hilum vs. elsewhere) contribute to the varied behavior of epithelial cells, depending on their address within the ovary.

At each ovulation the ovarian epithelium experiences injury by rupture, with the continuous layer of surface epithelium (and underlying tunica albuginea) sustaining repetitive damage. It is assumed that stem cells in the remaining surface epithelium are involved in repairing this rupture; murine studies have implicated stem/progenitor cells in the ovarian surface epithelium as central to this process [63]. Specifically, pulse-chase experiments using 5-bromodeoxyuridine and transgenic mice were able to show a population of long-term label-retaining cells in the surface epithelial layer. Although dormant before ovulation, these cells activated and began replicating at the follicular margins soon afterward, indicating that these cells were contributing to repair and remodeling processes.

Mesenchymal cells in the tunica albuginea of the adult ovary can undergo a mesenchymal–epithelial transition into ovarian surface epithelium cells, which differentiate sequentially into primitive granulosa and germ cells. These structures have now been shown to assemble in deeper ovarian cortex to form new follicles, replacing older (atretic) primary follicles. Such follicular renewal has been reported in rat ovaries, and human oocytes can differentiate from ovarian surface epithelium in fetal ovaries *in vivo* and from adult ovaries *in vitro*. Thus the pool of primary follicles

Bioscience Reports (2019) **39** BSR20190805
https://doi.org/10.1042/BSR20190805

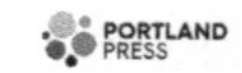

in adult human ovaries does not represent a static, but rather a dynamic, population of differentiating and regressing structures [6].

What signaling events might call progenitor cells (or stem cells) forward within the ovary to activate a post-ovulatory local tissue injury repair? And which markers seem most relevant to study in this regard? It has been suggested that WNT/β-catenin are involved in this process by differentiation of progenitor cells in the ovarian surface epithelium [64]. Specifically, transgenic mice with a β-catenin/TCF (T-cell factor)-responsive lacZ reporter gene were studied to help identify WNT-activated cells. Interestingly, lacZ expression occurred in the undifferentiated gonad, but after sex determination, expression was limited to the female gonad—a pattern agreeing with the membranous localization of β-catenin in embryonic murine gonads [65]. Furthermore, this ovarian surface epithelium cell gene expression declined after birth to a population of just 0.2% of the total surface epithelial cell population. This decline was not secondary to apoptosis or reduced proliferation, but rather from lacZ-positive cells differentiating into lacZ-negative cells. Thus, lacZ-positive cells (active β-catenin/TCF signaling) in the ovarian surface epithelium seem to act as stem cells, capable of contributing to repairing ovarian surface microtrauma. In addition, WNT4 and RSPO1 up-regulate the adult stem cell marker LGR5 in developing mouse ovaries, again suggesting that this pathway directs stem cell activity at the ovary surface [66]. A population of cells has been isolated by flow cytometry from the ovarian surface epithelium of adult mice [67], expressing high levels of mRNA for the hematopoietic stem cell marker lymphocyte antigen 6 complex, locus A (LY6A). Constituting only 2% of the total surface epithelial cell population, this LY6A+ subpopulation is detectable after approximately 4 weeks. In contrast, LY6A− cells proliferated much earlier, in the first 7 days. Moreover, a process seen in stem cells known as spheroid formation was higher in LY6A+ cells compared with other surface epithelial cells. LY6A+ cells existed in the surface layer and were not in direct contact with any other ovarian structures such as follicle walls or corpora lutea. Such cells appeared more cuboidal compared with the remaining surface epithelial cells, and additionally, oocytes of primordial follicles were LY6A+. Since there is increasing evidence for the existence of GSCs on the surface of murine ovaries [38], any LY6A+ cells detected in ovarian tissue sections could be GSCs rather than progenitor cells/stem cells of ovarian surface epithelium.

Cells have been identified in the hilar region of postnatal mouse ovaries which show classical stem cell characteristics such as expression of ALDH1 (aldehyde dehydrogenase 1), LGR5, CD133 (cluster of differentiation 133), CK6B (cytokeratin 6B), and LEF1 (lymphoid enhancer-binding factor 1), as well as long-term survival/proliferation and spheroid formation in culture [61]. Importantly, the previously noted pulse-chase experiments (using 5-bromodeoxyuridine labeling) have provided evidence that these cells are specifically activated to repair the rupture/injury at the surface of the ovary following ovulation, apparently to seal off the irregular surface at the site of ovulation [62]. LGR5 expression was located on the surface and subsurface region in the fetal mouse ovary, although this was confined to the surface epithelium by postnatal d7 and in adult mice. Additional research will be needed to establish if LGR5+ cells are confined to specific epithelial areas of the ovarian hilum [61], or more widely distributed throughout the entire ovarian surface [66].

Human adult ovary research has shown that most (>75%) of surface epithelial cells express the known stem cell marker NANOG, secreted frizzled related protein 1 (SFRP1), LIM homeobox 9 (LHX9), and ALDH1A2, yet only 25% of ovarian surface epithelial cells were ALDH1A1+ [4]. Assuming these specialized cells are present in the adult human ovary, an important question which remains to be examined is this: Given what is currently known about surface markers, under what conditions might discrete signaling be produced to evoke differentiation of any precursor cell(s) to become functional *de novo* oocytes?

The platelet signaling milieu

Relevant parallels exist between wound healing and ovarian tissue repair following capsule rupture at ovulation, and some molecular signaling events which might be necessary to reverse the effects of reproductive aging seem congruent with changes occurring in tissue injury responses elsewhere [68,69]. The interaction between platelets and plasma proteins—notably fibrin formed from fibrinogen by thrombin—causes fibrin clot formation, itself a reservoir of growth factors. These are discharged into plasma from α-granules of platelets when they are activated during wound healing and tissue regeneration. Platelet α granules [70,71] contain numerous cell signaling moieties directly involved in tissue repair such as HGF, SDF-1, adenosine diphosphate, serotonin, and sphingosine-1-phosphate; these can promote survival signals for vascular endothelial cells and SMCs (smooth muscle cells) at sites of vascular injury [72–74]. Transforming growth factor β isoform 1 (TGF-β1) is of pivotal importance given its actions on cell proliferation, angiogenesis, and extracellular matrix deposition [75]. One application of this may be seen in improved endothelial regeneration observed following injection of platelet microparticles in a mouse carotid artery injury model [76]. Platelets are also known to influence certain progenitor cell actions following tissue insult. For example, SDF-1 secreted by activated platelets support CD34-positive progenitor cell recruitment to arterial thrombi and differentiation of endothelial progenitor cells *in vivo* [77]. In the setting of myocardial infarction, platelet-derived SDF-1 was related to the number of circulating progenitor cells and was associated with restoration of left ventricular function and an improved prognosis. Formation of circulating platelet/CD34+ progenitor cell co-aggregates has been reported in patients with acute coronary syndromes, which was associated with a significantly decreased myocardial infarct size and better left ventricular function, as seen with cardiac magnetic resonance imaging at a 3-month follow-up [78–80]. However, platelet-induced differentiation of CD34-positive progenitors into mature foam cells and endothelial cells has been described in an *in vitro* co-culture system [81], which may be of particular relevance for development of atherosclerotic vascular lesions. Injection of autologous PRP (platelet-rich plasma) may terminate or even reverse the progress of early disc disease in the rabbit, which may be associated with the role of multiple growth factors of PRP in regulating cell function, improving tissue microenvironment, and/or modulating tissue regeneration [82].

Such platelet-derived growth factors are large, hydrophilic molecules with a molecular weight above 15 kDa. Unlikely to penetrate skin in sufficient quantities to be clinically significant [83], these growth factors must be injected directly into ovarian tissue to attain any meaningful therapeutic effect. Once deposited within the ovary, growth factor ligands have an opportunity to interact with receptors and regulators to influence cell differentiation outcomes (see Figure 2). An understanding of ovarian stem cell biology as outlined previously, and how this may be modulated should enhance understanding of ovary biology in general, and PRP actions in particular. For example, the growth factors produced from PRP represent a diverse group of regulatory proteins which attach to cell membrane receptors mediating important chemical messages. Via this interaction, they enable inter- and intracellular signaling pathways to govern cell growth, proliferation, and differentiation. Unlike hormones, these growth factors show quite circumscribed activity, physiologically relevant only in very close proximity to their release site. These local effects include mitogenesis, angiogenesis, chemotaxis, and formation of the extracellular matrix and even controlling release of other growth factors [83,84].

Previous research has revealed multiple critical roles of these growth factors and their receptors in embryonic and postnatal development. PDGF was originally identified in platelets and in serum as a mitogen for fibroblasts, SMCs and glia cells in culture. PDGF has since expanded to a family of dimers of at least four gene products, whose biological actions are mediated through two receptor tyrosine kinases. These products of activated platelets seem to act upon specific populations of progenitor cells that yield several different cell types with distinct functions in a variety of developmental processes. Given the wide scope of action, it is plausible that PRP elements might supply the requisite signal(s) needed to induce precursor or stem cell differentiation into a mature oocyte.

This inference finds support from earlier work which showed rescue from developmental arrest depends on PDGF (and other platelet-derived mediators like IGF-1), where these cytokines trigger DNA synthesis and cell-cycle specific proto-oncogenes *fos* and *myc* [85] with entry into mitosis within 24 h [86,87]. Studies on PDGF have led to an understanding of how cells detect a gradient of attractant and crawl toward it [88]. Guidance of cell migration during ovarian development shows mechanistic overlap with axon pathfinding, with some guidance cues used for both axon pathfinding and cell migration [89]. This role of PDGF in guiding cell migration has been investigated directly *in vivo* [90]. The migration of somatic (border) cells in Drosophila was chosen as model for directional migration in a genetically tractable system, where cells were noted to delaminate from the anterior follicular epithelium and move toward the oocyte. Upon arrival at the egg, they migrate a short distance dorsally toward the germinal vesicle, a PDGF-modulated process which is critical for female fertility [91].

Clinical applications: intraovarian PRP

The breakthrough application of PRP in a reproductive context was an innovation first outlined only a few years ago [92], when a group of poor prognosis infertility patients received intraovarian injection of PRP followed by IVF with non-donor oocytes. Using autologous (conventional, non-activated) PRP in this setting was considered a logical extension of the beneficial tissue effects following standard PRP administration as documented in other clinical settings [93–95]. The rationale here was to concentrate and provide the previously described growth factors directly to a new target tissue—the adult human ovary.

Numerous cytokines, chemokines, and growth factors (e.g., hepatocyte growth factor, stromal-derived growth factor-1) have been identified as platelet products. Such platelet-derived mediators induce and modulate activation of fibroblasts and recruitment of leukocytes, neutrophils, and macrophages, resulting in elimination of dead cells and cellular debris [96]. Platelet-released factors also control proliferation and migration of other cells essential to tissue repair [72]. Angiogenesis in damaged tissue, another pivotal mechanism for tissue repair, is also regulated by platelets via release of numerous pro- and anti-angiogenic mediators upon platelet activation [97].

Bioscience Reports (2019) **39** BSR20190805
https://doi.org/10.1042/BSR20190805

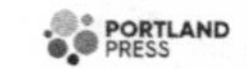

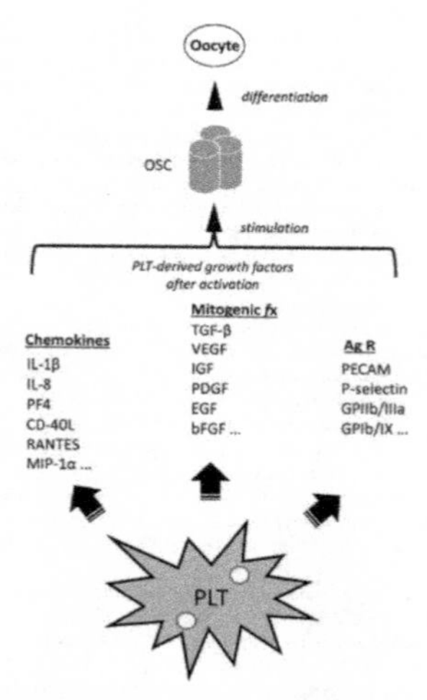

Figure 2. Proposed mechanism of action for alteration of adult ovarian function by application of activated PRP
Autologous activated PRP sample generates an enriched platelet (PLT) substrate collected by peripheral venipuncture. PLT combination with calcium gluconate achieves activation of α granules [red circles], which subsequently initiates release of at least three classes of molecular mediators. These include chemokines such as Interleukin-1β (IL-1β), a central inflammatory mediator involved in cell proliferation, differentiation, and apoptosis; Interleukin-8 (IL-8, also known as neutrophil chemotactic factor) which coordinates migration toward sites of injury or infection and is a promoter of angiogenesis and improved tissue perfusion; Platelet factor 4 (PF4), a versatile chemotactic protein with high affinity for heparin, involved in platelet aggregation and selective antimicrobial activity; Ligand of CD40 (CD-40L), a potent inducer of inflammatory processes by enhancing interactions among platelets, leukocytes, and endothelium; a protein known as Regulated after Activation of Normal T-cell Expressed and Secreted (RANTES), itself a useful marker for PLT activation which strongly attracts monocytes; Macrophage inflammatory protein 1-α (MIP-1α), which conditionally triggers migration and signaling cascades to mediate cell survival and proliferation; Platelet-associated cellular mitogens include TGF-β, which activates different downstream substrates and regulatory proteins inducing transcription of multiple target genes for differentiation, chemotaxis, proliferation and activation of immune system cells; Vascular endothelial growth factor (VEGF), a signal protein stimulating blood vessel formation; Insulin like growth factors (IGFs) a group of proteins with close homology to insulin required for cell stimulation and communication with the local environment; Platelet derived growth factor (PDGF), critical in growth of blood vessels from extant nearby capillaries, mitogenesis and proliferation of mesenchymal cells including fibroblasts, osteoblasts, tenocytes, vascular SMCs and mesenchymal stem cells; epidermal growth factor (EGF), a central element in cellular proliferation, differentiation, and survival; Basic fibroblast growth factor (bFGF), a mediator with broad mitogenic and cell survival activities, and is involved in a variety of biological processes, including embryonic development, cell growth, morphogenesis, tissue repair, tumor growth and invasion function. Platelet expressed antigens include Platelet endothelial cell adhesion molecule (PECAM), which plays a key role in removing aged neutrophils from circulation; P-selectin which contributes to initial recruitment of leukocytes to injury sites during inflammation; Glycoprotein IIb/IIIa, part of the integrin complex found on platelets aiding in platelet activation; and Glycoprotein Ib and IX (GPIb/IX) which binds von Willebrand factor, allowing platelet adhesion and platelet plug formation at sites of vascular injury. PRP is placed inside the adult ovary (by direct ultrasound-guided needle injection) thus permitting these signaling elements access to ovarian stem cells (OSCs) as discussed by Johnson et al. (2004). PLT-derived moieties then trigger or enable differentiation of these OSCs. Subsequently, reduced serum FSH and/or higher post-treatment levels of serum AMH have been observed clinically, consistent with improved or 're-potentiated' ovarian function.

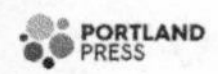

When autologous-activated PRP is injected into human ovarian tissue, several early observations have been noted with respect to organ function over time. Day 3 FSH/estradiol (and to a lesser extent, serum AMH) have been shown to improve following activated PRP injection into ovarian tissue [98]. While serum AMH may transiently decline (and/or FSH may briefly increase) within 2–4 weeks of intraovarian PRP injection for some patients, other recipients of ovarian autologous-activated PRP appear to skip this step and directly manifest an immediate improvement in reserve markers. The former pattern could be explained by a functional model, whereby the ovary sustains a temporary insult secondary to needle injection microtrauma associated with delivering the autologous activated PRP to the ovary. Why some patients do not demonstrate this sequence after the ovarian PRP procedure remains unknown, although this variance could be simply related to surgical/anatomical differences among PRP study patients. Additional analysis will be required to develop a more complete understanding of this recently noted ovarian tissue phenomenon.

Against this background, investigators are presented with many pieces of an unclear puzzle. The regenerative and repair processes instigated by PRP in somatic tissues remain only partially understood. PRP effects in the adult human ovary are even less known. If ovarian stem cells are indeed present, what is the risk that activated PRP might trigger tumorigenic or malignant transformations? Thus far, no adverse effects have been noted from international work using ovarian PRP, but clinical progress must be mindful of the possibility of untoward outcomes. Certainly for some poor-prognosis IVF patients, intraovarian injection of activated autologous PRP has been found to be beneficial, as frozen blastocysts and even pregnancies have been achieved without reliance on donor oocytes [98,99].

From a PRP sample preparation perspective, the role of platelet activation is likely to be important as this facilitates (and optimizes) platelet growth factor release. Commonly used techniques for platelet activation include addition of ADP [100], thrombin [101], collagen [102], Ca^{++} chloride [103], Ca^{++} gluconate [98,104], or combinations of these reagents [105–109]. Typically, platelet concentration in PRP may be up to ten times greater than ambient platelet concentration in peripheral circulation [83]. While early experience with ovarian PRP has been described [98,99], the exact mechanism of action, the role of platelet activation, and best clinical protocol have not been precisely established. For example, what platelet-derived mediators are most important in altering (improving) ovarian capacity after ovarian exposure to PRP? Do resident ovarian stem cells receive differentiation signals from PRP products as a contribution to this effect, and if so, how? Alternatively, do any oocytes harvested from PRP-treated ovaries represent a latent reserve population of dormant follicles which become eligible for recruitment following intrastromal injection of PRP? Ongoing work is designed to address each of these issues.

Conclusion

Advanced maternal age and its associated poor ovarian reserve cannot be reliably corrected simply by gonadotropin stimulation alone. The matter of existence of adult ovarian GSCs is clearly central to activated PRP use in a reproductive setting, yet the debate is far from settled [110]. There may be sufficient evidence to include GSCs in the postnatal folliculogenesis model [111] although the traditional dogma of non-renewable, limited oocyte stores also retains serious support [112]. It could be that any putative adult ovarian GSCs are really just dedifferentiated cells which then develop as germ cells under specific *in vitro* conditions [113], as dedifferentiation has been noted in other cell types [114]. Whether or not adult ovarian GSCs represent true oogonial stem cells, and the question of whether they are clinically relevant may receive at least a partial answer from early data on IVF following intraovarian PRP dosing [98,99]. Unless some procedure can be developed to restore the native oocyte pool, continued reliance on donor oocytes for IVF will be necessary. What is has been noted from clinical work with intraovarian PRP may be regarded as an echo of ancestral growth factor functions, iterated in related sets of morphogenetic processes during evolutionary development [115]. Our understanding of the activated PRP substrate, its derivative growth factors, putative receptor targets, differentiation regulators, as well as other aspects of this innovative approach are at a nascent stage [116]. It is plausible that any improved ovarian function observed after exposure of adult ovarian tissue to PRP components is merely a manifestation of precursor cell differentiation [117,118], evoked by still poorly understood growth signals of platelet origin.

Competing Interests

E.S.S. holds a provisional U.S. patent for process and treatment using ovarian PRP.

Funding

The authors declare that there are no sources of funding to be acknowledged.

Bioscience Reports (2019) **39** BSR20190805
https://doi.org/10.1042/BSR20190805

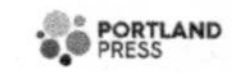

Author Contribution

Both authors contributed equally to this work.

Abbreviations

ALDH1, aldehyde dehydrogenase 1; BMP, bone morphogenetic protein; CD133, cluster of differentiation 133; DPPA3, developmental pluripotency associated 3; GFP, green fluorescent protein; GSC, germline stem cell; IFITM3, interferon-induced transmembrane protein 3; LY6A, lymphocyte antigen 6 complex, locus A; PDGF, platelet-derived growth factor; PGC, primordial germ cell; PRP, platelet-rich plasma; SMC, smooth muscle cell; Sox2, SRY box 2; SSEA, stage-specific embryonic antigen; Stra8, stimulated by retinoic acid 8; TCF, T-cell factor; TGF-β, transforming growth factor β; Utf1, undifferentiated embryonic cell transcript factor-1; VSEL, very small embryonic-like stem cell; Zfp296, zinc finger protein 296.

References

1 Sills, E.S., Alper, M.M. and Walsh, A.P. (2009) Ovarian reserve screening in infertility: practical applications and theoretical directions for research. *Eur. J. Obstet. Gynecol. Reprod. Biol.* **146**, 30–36, https://doi.org/10.1016/j.ejogrb.2009.05.008

2 Hsueh, A.J., Kawamura, K., Cheng, Y. and Fauser, B.C. (2015) Intraovarian control of early folliculogenesis. *Endocr. Rev.* **36**, 1–24, https://doi.org/10.1210/er.2014-1020

3 Robin, C., Ottersbach, K., de Bruijn, M., Ma, X., van der Horn, K. and Dzierzak, E. (2003) Developmental origins of hematopoietic stem cells. *Oncol. Res.* **13**, 315–321, https://doi.org/10.3727/096504003108748519

4 Hummitzsch, K., Anderson, R.A., Wilhelm, D., Wu, J., Telfer, E.E., Russell, D.L. et al. (2015) Stem cells, progenitor cells, and lineage decisions in the ovary. *Endocr. Rev.* **36**, 65–91, https://doi.org/10.1210/er.2014-1079

5 Guigon, C.J. and Cohen-Tannoudji, M. (2011) Reconsidering the roles of female germ cells in ovarian development and folliculogenesis. *Biol. Aujourdhui* **205**, 223–233, https://doi.org/10.1051/jbio/2011022

6 Bukovsky, A., Caudle, M.R., Svetlikova, M., Wimalasena, J., Ayala, M.E. and Dominguez, R. (2005) Oogenesis in adult mammals, including humans: a review. *Endocrine* **26**, 301–316, https://doi.org/10.1385/ENDO:26:3:301

7 Parte, S., Bhartiya, D., Telang, J., Daithankar, V., Salvi, V., Zaveri, K. et al. (2011) Detection, characterization, and spontaneous differentiation *in vitro* of very small embryonic-like putative stem cells in adult mammalian ovary. *Stem Cells Dev.* **20**, 1451–1464, https://doi.org/10.1089/scd.2010.0461

8 Virant-Klun, I., Zech, N., Rozman, P., Vogler, A., Cvjeticanin, B., Klemenc, P. et al. (2008) Putative stem cells with an embryonic character isolated from the ovarian surface epithelium of women with no naturally present follicles and oocytes. *Differentiation* **76**, 843–856, https://doi.org/10.1111/j.1432-0436.2008.00268.x

9 Motta, P.M. and Makabe, S. (1986) Elimination of germ cells during differentiation of the human ovary: an electron microscopic study. *Eur. J. Obstet. Gynecol. Reprod. Biol.* **22**, 271–286, https://doi.org/10.1016/0028-2243(86)90115-2

10 Kerr, J.B., Duckett, R., Myers, M., Britt, K.L., Mladenovska, T. and Findlay, J.K. (2006) Quantification of healthy follicles in the neonatal and adult mouse ovary: evidence for maintenance of primordial follicle supply. *Reproduction* **132**, 95–109, https://doi.org/10.1530/rep.1.01128

11 White, Y.A., Woods, D.C., Takai, Y., Ishihara, O., Seki, H. and Tilly, J.L. (2012) Oocyte formation by mitotically active germ cells purified from ovaries of reproductive-age women. *Nat. Med.* **18**, 413–421, https://doi.org/10.1038/nm.2669

12 Zuckerman, S. (1951) The number of oocytes in the mature ovary. *Recent Prog. Horm. Res.* **6**, 63–109

13 Johnson, J., Canning, J., Kaneko, T., Pru, J.K. and Tilly, J.L. (2004) Germline stem cells and follicular renewal in the postnatal mammalian ovary. *Nature* **428**, 145–150, https://doi.org/10.1038/nature02316

14 Zou, K., Yuan, Z., Yang, Z. et al. (2009) Production of offspring from a germline stem cell line derived from neonatal ovaries. *Nat. Cell Biol.* **11**, 631–636, https://doi.org/10.1038/ncb1869

15 Zhou, L., Wang, L., Kang, J.X. et al. (2014) Production of fat-1 transgenic rats using a post-natal female germline stem cell line. *Mol. Hum. Reprod.* **20**, 271–281, https://doi.org/10.1093/molehr/gat081

16 Johnson, J., Bagley, J., Skaznik-Wikiel, M. et al. (2005) Oocyte generation in adult mammalian ovaries by putative germ cells in bone marrow and peripheral blood. *Cell* **122**, 303–315, https://doi.org/10.1016/j.cell.2005.06.031

17 Eggan, K., Jurga, S., Gosden, R., Min, I.M. and Wagers, A.J. (2006) Ovulated oocytes in adult mice derive from non-circulating germ cells. *Nature* **441**, 1109–1114, https://doi.org/10.1038/nature04929

18 Lee, H.J., Selesniemi, K., Niikura, Y. et al. (2007) Bone marrow transplantation generates immature oocytes and rescues long-term fertility in a preclinical mouse model of chemotherapy-induced premature ovarian failure. *J. Clin. Oncol.* **25**, 3198–3204, https://doi.org/10.1200/JCO.2006.10.3028

19 Notarianni, E. (2011) Reinterpretation of evidence advanced for neo-oogenesis in mammals, in terms of a finite oocyte reserve. *J. Ovarian Res.* **4**, 1, https://doi.org/10.1186/1757-2215-4-1

20 Zulli, A., Rai, S., Buxton, B.F., Burrell, L.M. and Hare, D.L. (2008) Co-localization of angiotensin-converting enzyme 2-, octomer-4- and CD34-positive cells in rabbit atherosclerotic plaques. *Exp. Physiol.* **93**, 564–569, https://doi.org/10.1113/expphysiol.2007.040204

21 Brännström, M., Mayrhofer, G. and Robertson, S.A. (1993) Localization of leukocyte subsets in the rat ovary during the periovulatory period. *Biol. Reprod.* **48**, 277–286, https://doi.org/10.1095/biolreprod48.2.277

22 Best, C.L., Pudney, J., Welch, W.R., Burger, N. and Hill, J.A. (1996) Localization and characterization of white blood cell populations within the human ovary throughout the menstrual cycle and menopause. *Hum. Reprod.* **11**, 790–797, https://doi.org/10.1093/oxfordjournals.humrep.a019256

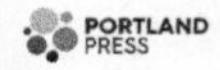

23 Samy, E.T., Parker, L.A., Sharp, C.P. and Tung, K.S. (2005) Continuous control of autoimmune disease by antigen-dependent polyclonal CD4+CD25+ regulatory T cells in the regional lymph node. *J. Exp. Med.* **202**, 771–781, https://doi.org/10.1084/jem.20041033
24 Samy, E.T., Setiady, Y.Y., Ohno, K., Pramoonjago, P., Sharp, C. and Tung, K.S. (2006) The role of physiological self-antigen in the acquisition and maintenance of regulatory T-cell function. *Immunol. Rev.* **212**, 170–184, https://doi.org/10.1111/j.0105-2896.2006.00404.x
25 Alard, P., Thompson, C., Agersborg, S.S. et al. (2001) Endogenous oocyte antigens are required for rapid induction and progression of autoimmune ovarian disease following day-3 thymectomy. *J. Immunol.* **166**, 4363–4369, https://doi.org/10.4049/jimmunol.166.7.4363
26 Reizel, Y., Itzkovitz, S., Adar, R. et al. (2012) Cell lineage analysis of the mammalian female germline. *PLoS Genet.* **8**, e1002477, https://doi.org/10.1371/journal.pgen.1002477
27 Henderson, S.A. and Edwards, R.G. (1968) Chiasma frequency and maternal age in mammals. *Nature* **218**, 22–28, https://doi.org/10.1038/218022a0
28 Pacchiarotti, J., Maki, C., Ramos, T. et al. (2010) Differentiation potential of germ line stem cells derived from the postnatal mouse ovary. *Differentiation* **79**, 159–170, https://doi.org/10.1016/j.diff.2010.01.001
29 Zhang, Y., Yang, Z., Yang, Y. et al. (2011) Production of transgenic mice by random recombination of targeted genes in female germline stem cells. *J. Mol. Cell Biol.* **3**, 132–141, https://doi.org/10.1093/jmcb/mjq043
30 Zhang, Y. and Wu, J. (2009) Molecular cloning and characterization of a new gene, Oocyte-G1. *J. Cell. Physiol.* **218**, 75–83, https://doi.org/10.1002/jcp.21569
31 Imudia, A.N., Wang, N., Tanaka, Y., White, Y.A., Woods, D.C. and Tilly, J.L. (2013) Comparative gene expression profiling of adult mouse ovary-derived oogonial stem cells supports a distinct cellular identity. *Fertil. Steril.* **100**, 1451–1458, https://doi.org/10.1016/j.fertnstert.2013.06.036
32 Park, E.S., Woods, D.C. and Tilly, J.L. (2013) Bone morphogenetic protein 4 promotes mammalian oogonial stem cell differentiation via Smad1/5/8 signaling. *Fertil. Steril.* **100**, 1468–1475, https://doi.org/10.1016/j.fertnstert.2013.07.1978
33 Lawson, K.A., Dunn, N.R., Roelen, B.A. et al. (1999) Bmp4 is required for the generation of primordial germ cells in the mouse embryo. *Genes Dev.* **13**, 424–436, https://doi.org/10.1101/gad.13.4.424
34 Childs, A.J., Kinnell, H.L., Collins, C.S. et al. (2010) BMP signaling in the human fetal ovary is developmentally regulated and promotes primordial germ cell apoptosis. *Stem Cells* **28**, 1368–1378, https://doi.org/10.1002/stem.440
35 Le Bouffant, R., Souquet, B., Duval, N. et al. (2011) Msx1 and Msx2 promote meiosis initiation. *Development* **138**, 5393–5402, https://doi.org/10.1242/dev.068452
36 Abban, G. and Johnson, J. (2009) Stem cell support of oogenesis in the human. *Hum. Reprod.* **24**, 2974–2978, https://doi.org/10.1093/humrep/dep281
37 Castrillon, D.H., Quade, B.J., Wang, T.Y., Quigley, C. and Crum, C.P. (2000) The human VASA gene is specifically expressed in the germ cell lineage. *Proc. Natl Acad. Sci. U.S.A.* **97**, 9585–9590, https://doi.org/10.1073/pnas.160274797
38 Zou, K., Hou, L., Sun, K., Xie, W. and Wu, J. (2011) Improved efficiency of female germline stem cell purification using fragilis-based magnetic bead sorting. *Stem Cells Dev.* **20**, 2197–2204, https://doi.org/10.1089/scd.2011.0091
39 Wang, H., Jiang, M., Bi, H. et al. (2014) Conversion of female germline stem cells from neonatal and prepubertal mice into pluripotent stem cells. *J. Mol. Cell Biol.* **6**, 164–171, https://doi.org/10.1093/jmcb/mju004
40 Xie, W., Wang, H. and Wu, J. (2014) Similar morphological and molecular signatures shared by female and male germline stem cells. *Sci. Rep.* **4**, 5580, https://doi.org/10.1038/srep05580
41 Møllgård, K., Jespersen, A., Lutterodt, M.C., Yding Andersen, C., Høyer, P.E. and Byskov, A.G. (2010) Human primordial germ cells migrate along nerve fibers and Schwann cells from the dorsal hind gut mesentery to the gonadal ridge. *Mol. Hum. Reprod.* **16**, 621–631, https://doi.org/10.1093/molehr/gaq052
42 Bendel-Stenzel, M., Anderson, R., Heasman, J. and Wylie, C. (1998) The origin and migration of primordial germ cells in the mouse. *Semin. Cell Dev. Biol.* **9**, 393–400, https://doi.org/10.1006/scdb.1998.0204
43 De Felici, M. (2010) Germ stem cells in the mammalian adult ovary: considerations by a fan of the primordial germ cells. *Mol. Hum. Reprod.* **16**, 632–636, https://doi.org/10.1093/molehr/gaq006
44 Shin, D.M., Zuba-Surma, E.K., Wu, W., Ratajczak, J., Wysoczynski, M., Ratajczak, M.Z. et al. (2009) Novel epigenetic mechanisms that control pluripotency and quiescence of adult bone marrow-derived Oct4(þ) very small embryonic-like stem cells. *Leukemia* **23**, 2042–2051, https://doi.org/10.1038/leu.2009.153
45 Kucia, M., Maj, M., Mierzejewska, K., Shin, D.M., Ratajczak, J. and Ratajczak, M.Z. (2013) Challenging dogmas - or how much evidence is necessary to claim that there is a direct developmental and functional link between the primordial germ cell (PGC) lineage and hematopoiesis. *Blood* **122**, 21
46 Havens, A.M., Shiozawa, Y., Jung, Y., Sun, H., Wang, J., McGee, S. et al. (2013) Human very small embryonic-like cells generate skeletal structures, *in vivo*. *Stem Cells Dev.* **22**, 622–630, https://doi.org/10.1089/scd.2012.0327
47 Wojakowski, W., Ratajczak, M.Z. and Tendera, M. (2010) Mobilization of very small embryonic-like stem cells in acute coronary syndromes and stroke. *Herz* **35**, 467–472, https://doi.org/10.1007/s00059-010-3389-0
48 Sovalat, H., Scrofani, M., Eidenschenk, A., Pasquet, S., Rimelen, V. and Hénon, P. (2011) Identification and isolation from either adult human bone marrow or G-CSF-mobilized peripheral blood of CD34(+)/CD133(+)/CXCR4(+)/Lin(-)CD45(-) cells, featuring morphological, molecular, and phenotypic characteristics of very small embryonic-like (VSEL) stem cells. *Exp. Hematol.* **39**, 495–505
49 Drukala, J., Paczkowska, E., Kucia, M., Młyńska, E., Krajewski, A., Machaliński, B. et al. (2012) Stem cells, including a population of very small embryonic-like stem cells, are mobilized into peripheral blood in patients after skin burn injury. *Stem Cell Rev.* **8**, 184–194, https://doi.org/10.1007/s12015-011-9272-4
50 Bhartiya, D., Anand, S., Patel, H. and Parte, S. (2017) Making gametes from alternate sources of stem cells: past, present and future. *Reprod. Biol. Endocrinol.* **15**, 89, https://doi.org/10.1186/s12958-017-0308-8

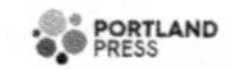

51 Byskov, A.G., Høyer, P.E., Yding Andersen, C., Kristensen, S.G., Jespersen, A. and Møllgård, K. (2011) No evidence for the presence of oogonia in the human ovary after their final clearance during the first two years of life. *Hum. Reprod.* **26**, 2129–2139, https://doi.org/10.1093/humrep/der145
52 Bhartiya, D., Unni, S., Parte, S. and Anand, S. (2013) Very small embryonic-like stem cells: implications in reproductive biology. *Biomed. Res. Int.* **2013**, 682326, https://doi.org/10.1155/2013/682326
53 Ratajczak, M.Z., Zuba-Surma, E., Wojakowski, W., Suszynska, M., Mierzejewska, K., Liu, R. et al. (2014) Very small embryonic-like stem cells (VSELs) represent a real challenge in stem cell biology: recent pros and cons in the midst of a lively debate. *Leukemia* **28**, 473–484, https://doi.org/10.1038/leu.2013.255
54 Bhartiya, D., Hinduja, I., Patel, H. and Bhilawadikar, R. (2014) Making gametes from pluripotent stem cells–a promising role for very small embryonic-like stem cells. *Reprod. Biol. Endocrinol.* **12**, 114, https://doi.org/10.1186/1477-7827-12-114
55 Ratajczak, M. (2012) Igf2-H19, an imprinted tandem gene, is an important regulator of embryonic development, a guardian of proliferation of adult pluripotent stem cells, a regulator of longevity, and a 'passkey' to cancerogenesis. *Folia Histochem. Cytobiol.* **50**, 171–179, https://doi.org/10.5603/FHC.2012.0026
56 Monti, M., Imberti, B., Bianchi, N., Pezzotta, A., Morigi, M., Del Fante, C. et al. (2017) A novel method for isolation of pluripotent stem cells from human umbilical cord blood. *Stem Cells Dev.* **26**, 1258–1269, https://doi.org/10.1089/scd.2017.0012
57 Binelli, M. and Murphy, B.D. (2010) Coordinated regulation of follicle development by germ and somatic cells. *Reprod. Fertil. Dev.* **22**, 1–12, https://doi.org/10.1071/RD09218
58 Byskov, A.G. (1986) Differentiation of mammalian embryonic gonad. *Physiol. Rev.* **66**, 71–117, https://doi.org/10.1152/physrev.1986.66.1.71
59 Auersperg, N., Wong, A.S., Choi, K.C., Kang, S.K. and Leung, P.C. (2001) Ovarian surface epithelium: biology, endocrinology, and pathology. *Endocr. Rev.* **22**, 255–288
60 Hummitzsch, K., Irving-Rodgers, H.F., Hatzirodos, N. et al. (2013) A new model of development of the mammalian ovary and follicles. *PLoS ONE* **8**, e55578, https://doi.org/10.1371/journal.pone.0055578
61 Rodgers, R.J. and Hummitzsch, K. (2014) *New Model of Formation of the Ovary*, Robinson Research Institute, **http://www.youtube.com/watch?v=1097DtAyaDc**
62 Kenngott, R.A., Vermehren, M., Ebach, K. and Sinowatz, F. (2013) The role of ovarian surface epithelium in folliculogenesis during fetal development of the bovine ovary: a histological and immunohistochemical study. *Sex Dev.* **7**, 180–195, https://doi.org/10.1159/000348881
63 Szotek, P.P., Chang, H.L., Brennand, K. et al. (2008) Normal ovarian surface epithelial label-retaining cells exhibit stem/progenitor cell characteristics. *Proc. Natl. Acad. Sci. U.S.A.* **105**, 12469–12473, https://doi.org/10.1073/pnas.0805012105
64 Usongo, M. and Farookhi, R. (2012) β-Catenin/Tcf-signaling appears to establish the murine ovarian surface epithelium (OSE) and remains active in selected postnatal OSE cells. *BMC Dev. Biol.* **12**, 17, https://doi.org/10.1186/1471-213X-12-17
65 Bernard, P., Fleming, A., Lacombe, A., Harley, V.R. and Vilain, E. (2008) Wnt4 inhibits β-catenin/TCF signalling by redirecting β-catenin to the cell membrane. *Biol. Cell* **100**, 167–177, https://doi.org/10.1042/BC20070072
66 Rastetter, R.H., Bernard, P., Palmer, J.S. et al. (2014) Marker genes identify three somatic cell types in the fetal mouse ovary. *Dev. Biol.* **394**, 242–252, https://doi.org/10.1016/j.ydbio.2014.08.013
67 Gamwell, L.F., Collins, O. and Vanderhyden, B.C. (2012) The mouse ovarian surface epithelium contains a population of LY6A (SCA-1) expressing progenitor cells that are regulated by ovulation-associated factors. *Biol. Reprod.* **87**, 80
68 Martin, P. (1997) Wound healing—aiming for perfect skin regeneration. *Science* **276**, 75–81, https://doi.org/10.1126/science.276.5309.75
69 Hensley, K. and Floyd, R.A. (2002) Reactive oxygen species and protein oxidation in aging: a look back, a look ahead. *Arch. Biochem. Biophys.* **397**, 377–383, https://doi.org/10.1006/abbi.2001.2630
70 Mannaioni, P.F., Di Bello, G.M. and Masini, E. (1997) Platelets and inflammation: role of platelet-derived growth factor, adhesion molecules and histamine. *Inflamm. Res.* **46**, 4–18, https://doi.org/10.1007/PL00000158
71 Anitua, E., Andia, I., Ardanza, B., Nurden, P. and Nurden, A. (2004) Autologous platelets as a source of proteins for healing and tissue regeneration. *Thromb. Haemost.* **91**, 4–15, https://doi.org/10.1160/TH03-07-0440
72 Crowley, S.T., Dempsey, E.C., Horwitz, K.B. and Horwitz, L.D. (1994) Platelet-induced vascular smooth muscle cell proliferation is modulated by the growth amplification factors serotonin and adenosine diphosphate. *Circulation* **90**, 1908–1918, https://doi.org/10.1161/01.CIR.90.4.1908
73 Pakala, R., Willerson, J.T. and Benedict, C.R. (1994) Mitogenic effect of serotonin on vascular endothelial cells. *Circulation* **90**, 1919–1926, https://doi.org/10.1161/01.CIR.90.4.1919
74 Hisano, N., Yatomi, Y., Satoh, K., Akimoto, S., Mitsumata, M., Fujino, M.A. et al. (1999) Induction and suppression of endothelial cell apoptosis by sphingolipids: a possible in vitro model for cell-cell interactions between platelets and endothelial cells. *Blood* **93**, 4293–4299
75 Lee, K.S., Wilson, J.J., Rabago, D.P., Baer, G.S., Jacobson, J.A. and Borrero, C.G. (2011) Musculoskeletal applications of platelet-rich plasma: fad or future? *AJR Am. J. Roentgenol.* **196**, 628–636, https://doi.org/10.2214/AJR.10.5975
76 Mause, S.F., Ritzel, E., Liehn, E.A., Hristov, M., Bidzhekov, K., Müller-Newen, G. et al. (2010) Platelet microparticles enhance the vasoregenerative potential of angiogenic early outgrowth cells after vascular injury. *Circulation* **122**, 495–506, https://doi.org/10.1161/CIRCULATIONAHA.109.909473
77 Stellos, K., Langer, H., Daub, K. et al. (2008) Platelet-derived stromal cell-derived factor-1 regulates adhesion and promotes differentiation of human CD34+ cells to endothelial progenitor cells. *Circulation* **117**, 206–215, https://doi.org/10.1161/CIRCULATIONAHA.107.714691
78 Stellos, K., Bigalke, B., Langer, H. et al. (2009) Expression of stromal-cell-derived factor-1 on circulating platelets is increased in patients with acute coronary syndrome and correlates with the number of CD34+ progenitor cells. *Eur. Heart J.* **30**, 584–593, https://doi.org/10.1093/eurheartj/ehn566
79 Geisler, T., Fekecs, L., Wurster, T. et al. (2012) Association of platelet-SDF-1 with hemodynamic function and infarct size using cardiac MR in patients with AMI. *Eur. J. Radiol.* **81**, e486–e490, https://doi.org/10.1016/j.ejrad.2011.06.019

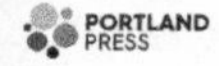

80 Stellos, K., Bigalke, B., Borst, O. et al. (2013) Circulating platelet-progenitor cell coaggregate formation is increased in patients with acute coronary syndromes and augments recruitment of CD34+ cells in the ischaemic microcirculation. *Eur. Heart J.* **34**, 2548–2556, https://doi.org/10.1093/eurheartj/eht131
81 Daub, K., Langer, H., Seizer, P. et al. (2006) Platelets induce differentiation of human CD34+ progenitor cells into foam cells and endothelial cells. *FASEB J.* **20**, 2559–2561, https://doi.org/10.1096/fj.06-6265fje
82 Hu, X., Wang, C. and Rui, Y. (2012) An experimental study on effect of autologous platelet-rich plasma on treatment of early intervertebral disc degeneration. *Zhongguo Xiu Fu Chong Jian Wai Ke Za Zhi* **26**, 977–983
83 Fabi, S. and Sundaram, H. (2014) The potential of topical and injectable growth factors and cytokines for skin rejuvenation. *Facial Plast. Surg.* **30**, 157–171, https://doi.org/10.1055/s-0034-1372423
84 Babu, M. and Wells, A. (2001) Dermal-epidermal communication in wound healing. *Wounds* **13**, 183–189
85 Müller, R., Bravo, R., Burckhardt, J. and Curran, T. (1984) Induction of c-fos gene and protein by growth factors precedes activation of c-myc. *Nature* **312**, 716–720, https://doi.org/10.1038/312716a0
86 Pardee, A.B. (1989) G1 events and regulation of cell proliferation. *Science* **246**, 603–608, https://doi.org/10.1126/science.2683075
87 Larson, R.C., Ignotz, G.G. and Currie, W.B. (1992) Platelet derived growth factor (PDGF) stimulates development of bovine embryos during the fourth cell cycle. *Development* **115**, 821–826
88 Lauffenburger, D.A. and Horwitz, A.F. (1996) Cell migration. *Cell* **84**, 359–369, https://doi.org/10.1016/S0092-8674(00)81280-5
89 Wu, Y.C. and Horvitz, H.R. (1998) C. elegans phagocytosis and cell-migration protein CED-5 is similar to human DOCK180. *Nature* **392**, 501–504, https://doi.org/10.1038/33163
90 Duchek, P., Somogyi, K., Jékely, G., Beccari, S. and Rørth, P. (2001) Guidance of cell migration by the *Drosophila* PDGF/VEGF receptor. *Cell* **107**, 17–26, https://doi.org/10.1016/S0092-8674(01)00502-5
91 Montell, D.J., Rørth, P. and Spradling, A.C. (1992) Slow border cells, a locus required for a developmentally regulated cell migration during oogenesis, encodes *Drosophila* C/EBP. *Cell* **71**, 51–62, https://doi.org/10.1016/0092-8674(92)90265-E
92 Pantos, K., Nitsos, N., Kokkali, G., Vaxevanoglu, T., Markomichaki, C., Pantou, A. et al. (2016) Ovarian rejuvenation and folliculogenesis reactivation in peri-menopausal women after autologous platelet-rich plasma treatment. Abstracts, ESHRE 32nd Annual Meeting, Helsinki, Finland, 3–6 July 2016. *Hum. Reprod.*, p. i301
93 Bonilla Horcajo, C., Zurita Castillo, M. and Vaquero Crespo, J. (2018) Platelet-rich plasma-derived scaffolds increase the benefit of delayed mesenchymal stromal cell therapy after severe traumatic brain injury. *Cytotherapy* **20**, 314–321, https://doi.org/10.1016/j.jcyt.2017.11.012
94 Sánchez, M., Delgado, D., Pompei, O., Pérez, J.C., Sánchez, P., Garate, A. et al. (2018) Treating severe knee osteoarthritis with combination of intra-osseous and intra-articular infiltrations of platelet-rich plasma: an observational study. *Cartilage* 1947603518756462
95 Tawfik, A.A. and Osman, M.A.R. (2018) The effect of autologous activated platelet-rich plasma injection on female pattern hair loss: a randomized placebo-controlled study. *J. Cosmet. Dermatol.* **17**, 47–53, https://doi.org/10.1111/jocd.12357
96 Gurtner, G.C., Werner, S., Barrandon, Y. and Longaker, M.T. (2008) Wound repair and regeneration. *Nature* **453**, 314–321, https://doi.org/10.1038/nature07039
97 Stellos, K., Kopf, S., Paul, A., Marquardt, J.U., Gawaz, M., Huard, J. et al. (2010) Platelets in regeneration. *Semin. Thromb. Hemost.* **36**, 175–184, https://doi.org/10.1055/s-0030-1251502
98 Sills, E.S., Rickers, N.S., Li, X. and Palermo, G.D. (2018) First data on in vitro fertilization and blastocyst formation after intraovarian injection of calcium gluconate-activated autologous platelet rich plasma. *Gynecol. Endocrinol.* 1–5
99 Sfakianoudis, K., Simopoulou, M., Nitsos, N., Rapani, A., Pantou, A., Vaxevanoglou, T. et al. (2018) A case series on platelet-rich plasma revolutionary management of poor responder patients. *Gynecol. Obstet. Invest.* 1–8
100 Rinder, H.M., Bonan, J.M., Ault, K.A. and Smith, B.R. (1991) Activated and unactivated platelet adhesion to monocytes and neutrophils. *Blood* **78**, 1760–1769
101 Waselau, M., Sutter, W.W., Genovese, R.L. and Bertone, A.L. (2008) Intralesional injection of platelet-rich plasma followed by controlled exercise for treatment of midbody suspensory ligament desmitis in standardbred racehorses. *J. Am. Vet. Med. Assoc.* **232**, 1515–1520, https://doi.org/10.2460/javma.232.10.1515
102 Fufa, D., Shealy, B., Jacobson, M., Sherwin, K. and Murray, M.M. (2008) Activation of platelet-rich plasma using Type I collagen. *J. Oral Maxillofac. Surg.* **66**, 684–690, https://doi.org/10.1016/j.joms.2007.06.635
103 Vos, R.J., Weir, A., van Schie, H.T.M., Bierma-Zeinstra, S.M.A., Verhaar, J.A.N., Weinans, H. et al. (2010) Platelet-rich plasma injection for chronic Achilles tendinopathy: a randomized controlled trial. *JAMA* **303**, 144–149, https://doi.org/10.1001/jama.2009.1986
104 Kitoh, H., Kitakoji, T., Tsuchiya, H., Mitsuyama, H., Nakamura, H., Katoh, M. et al. (2004) Transplantation of marrow-derived mesenchymal stem cell and platelet-rich plasma during distraction osteogenesis: a preliminary result of three cases. *Bone* **35**, 892–898, https://doi.org/10.1016/j.bone.2004.06.013
105 Everts, P.A.M., Mahoney, C.B., Hoffmann, J.J.M.L., Schönberger, J.P., Box, H.A.M., Van Zundert, A. et al. (2006) Platelet-rich plasma preparation using three devices: implications for platelet activation and platelet growth factor release. *Growth Factors* **24**, 165–171, https://doi.org/10.1080/08977190600821327
106 Gandhi, A., Doumas, C., O'Connor, J.P., Parsons, J.R. and Lin, S.S. (2006) The effects of local platelet rich plasma delivery on diabetic fracture healing. *Bone* **38**, 540–546, https://doi.org/10.1016/j.bone.2005.10.019
107 Virchenko, O. and Aspenberg, P. (2006) How one platelet injection after tendon injury can lead to a stronger tendon after 4 weeks. *Acta Orthop.* **77**, 806–812, https://doi.org/10.1080/17453670610013033
108 Monteiro, S.O., Lepage, O.M. and Theoret, C.L. (2009) Effects of platelet-rich plasma on the repair of wounds on the distal aspect of the forelimb in horses. *Am. J. Vet. Res.* **70**, 277–282, https://doi.org/10.2460/ajvr.70.2.277

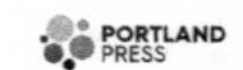

109 Zandim, B.M., de Souza, M.V., Magalhães, P.C., Benjamin, L., Maia, L., de Oliveira, A.C. et al. (2012) Platelet activation: Ultrastructure and morphometry in platelet-rich plasma of horses. *Pesq. Vet. Bras.* **32**, 83–92, https://doi.org/10.1590/S0100-736X2012000100014
110 Hanna, C.B. and Hennebold, J.D. (2014) Ovarian germline stem cells: an unlimited source of oocytes? *Fertil. Steril.* **101**, 20–30, https://doi.org/10.1016/j.fertnstert.2013.11.009
111 Dunlop, C.E. and Telfer, E.E. (2013) Anderson RA Ovarian stem cells—potential roles in infertility treatment and fertility preservation. *Maturitas* **76**, 279–283, https://doi.org/10.1016/j.maturitas.2013.04.017
112 Yuan, J., Zhang, D., Wang, L., Liu, M., Mao, J., Yin, Y. et al. (2013) No evidence for neo-oogenesis may link to ovarian senescence in adult monkey. *Stem Cells* **31**, 2538–2550, https://doi.org/10.1002/stem.1480
113 Lei, L. and Spradling, A.C. (2013) Female mice lack adult germ-line stem cells but sustain oogenesis using stable primordial follicles. *Proc. Nat. Acad. Sci. U.S.A.* **110**, 8585–9690, https://doi.org/10.1073/pnas.1306189110
114 Lee, S.T., Gong, S.P., Yum, K.E., Lee, E.J., Lee, C.H., Choi, J.H. et al. (2013) Transformation of somatic cells into stem cell-like cells under a stromal niche. *FASEB J.* **27**, 2644–2856, https://doi.org/10.1096/fj.12-223065
115 Betsholtz, C., Karlsson, L. and Lindahl, P. (2001) Developmental roles of platelet-derived growth factors. *Bioessays* **23**, 494–507, https://doi.org/10.1002/bies.1069
116 Powell, K. (2012) Egg-making stem cells found in adult ovaries. *Nature* **483**, 16, https://doi.org/10.1038/483016a
117 Sills, E.S., Li, X., Rickers, N.S., Wood, S.H. and Palermo, G.D. (2019) Metabolic and neurobehavioral response following intraovarian administration of autologous activated platelet rich plasma: first qualitative data. *Neuroendocrinol. Lett.* **39**, 427–433
118 Sills, E.S., Rickers, N.S., Svid, C.S., Rickers, J.M. and Wood, S.H. (2019) Normalized ploidy following 20 consecutive blastocysts with chromosomal error: healthy 46,XY pregnancy with IVF after intraovarian injection of autologous enriched platelet-derived growth factors. *Int. J. Mol. Cell. Med.* **8** (1), in press

Neuroendocrinology Letters Volume 39 No. 6 2018
ISSN: 0172-780X; ISSN-L: 0172-780X; Electronic/Online ISSN: 2354-4716
Web of Knowledge / Web of Science: Neuroendocrinol Lett
Pub Med / Medline: Neuro Endocrinol Lett

ORIGINAL ARTICLE

Metabolic and neurobehavioral response following intraovarian administration of autologous activated platelet rich plasma: First qualitative data

E. Scott Sills [1,2,4], Xiang Li [1,3], Natalie S. Rickers [1], Samuel H. Wood [4], Gianpiero D. Palermo [5]

1 Office for Reproductive Research, Center for Advanced Genetics; La Jolla, California USA
2 Applied Biotechnology Research Group, University of Westminster; London UK
3 Paralian Technology Inc., Mission Viejo, California USA
4 Gen 5 Fertility; La Jolla, California USA
5 Center for Reproductive Medicine & Infertility, Weill Medical College of Cornell University; New York NY USA

Correspondence to: Office for Reproductive Research, CAG at Gen 5 Fertility; 4150 Regents Park Row, Suite 300, La Jolla, California 92037 USA
FAX: +1 858-225-3535; E-MAIL: drsills@CAGivf.com

Submitted: 2018-10-20 *Accepted: 2018-11-02* *Published online: 2018-11-28*

Key words: **reproductive ageing; platelet rich plasma; ovary; sexual health; metabolism; rejuvenation**

Neuroendocrinol Lett 2018; **39**(6):427–433 **PMID:** 30796792 NEL390618A02 ©2018 Neuroendocrinology Letters • **www.nel.edu**

Abstract

OBJECTIVES: This work assessed sexual and neurobehavioral parameters after ovarian treatment with autologous PRP.
DESIGN: Questionnaire study.
MATERIAL AND METHODS: Patients receiving ovarian PRP injection (n=80) due to low ovarian reserve and/or at least 1 prior failed IVF cycle were sampled. Pre- and post-treatment levels in self-reported daily energy, sleep quality, skin tone/hair thickness/nail growth, cognitive clarity, menstrual pattern, cervical mucus/vaginal lubrication, libido, sexual activity, ability to achieve orgasm, and overall sexual experience were measured.
RESULTS: Mean±SD age and baseline BMI among patients were 45.5±6yrs and 25±5.1kg/m^2, respectively. Average weight loss after ovarian PRP was 1kg (p=0.028). After ovarian PRP, superior nail growth, skin tone, and hair thickness was observed by 46.3% of patients [95%CI=35%,57.8%]; the same ratio experienced increased "clarity of thinking" following the procedure. Irregular or absent menses affected 56.3% of patients at enrollment, and menses returned or cyclicity improved in 24.4% after treatment [95%CI=12.9%,39.5%]. Increased post-treatment vaginal lubrication/cervical mucus production was reported by 51.3% of women [95%CI=39.8%, 62.6%] accompanied by increased libido in 55% [95%CI=43.5%,66.2%]. More frequent sexual activity after ovarian PRP was noted from 46.3% of subjects [95%CI=35%, 57.8%] coinciding with a 45% improvement in overall sexual experience before vs. after ovarian PRP [95%CI=33.9%, 56.5%].
CONCLUSION: This investigation is the first to document responses across neurobehavioral and metabolic parameters after ovarian PRP. Injection of PRP-derived growth factors directly into ovarian tissue seems to enable a local signaling milieu favoring development of hormonally active ovarian elements, thus "re-potentiating" low or absent reserve.

INTRODUCTION

Platelets and their products (*i.e.*, platelet rich plasma, PRP) have well-established roles in managing thrombocytopenia, yet PRP also comprises many soluble mediators critical to coordinate cellular repair after tissue injury (Nurden, 2011). Closely linked to inflammatory signaling, PRP also modulates tissue regeneration, cell proliferation and migration, extracellular matrix remodeling, programmed cell death, differentiation, and angiogenesis (Gurtner *et al.*, 2008). Platelets are involved in the response to local tissue repair after capsular microtrauma in the adult human ovary after each ovulation, and likely contribute to overall organ function as well (Lacci & Dardik, 2010). Of note, the tissue regenerative effects of autologous PRP when applied to adult ovarian tissue have shown early promise in managing reduced reserve (Sfakianoudis *et al.*, 2018; Sills *et al.*, 2018). But independent of oocyte dynamics and IVF, what about broader, systemic responses following ovarian PRP? Here we report on selected effects of ovarian treatment with autologous PRP using a questionnaire-based qualitative research model.

MATERIAL AND METHODS

A retrospective chart review was performed to identify women who received autologous PRP to one or both ovaries at a single center, designed as an assessment extension for subjects who enrolled in registered clinical trial NCT03178695 (U.S. NLM, 2017). In brief, dosing consisted of fresh isolation of substrate followed by injection of activated PRP into ovarian stroma, as previously described.[4] Ovarian PRP treatments were performed at a single center, by one clinician using uniform equipment for all cases.

Patient and public involvement

A multidisciplinary team developed a 30-item research questionnaire, derived from the standardized Female Sexual Function Index (Crisp *et al.*, 2015) (see Table 1) Additional items were included based on redacted emails sent to clinic staff from patients after completing ovarian PRP. Queries were distributed by email invitation to those who underwent ovarian PRP procedure during a 16-month interval beginning April 2017. The questionnaire was configured electronically for secure internet access; there was no cost to participate and patients received nothing of value in exchange for contributing to the study. Participants were not able to access cumulative results until all data were received upon closure of the study. When the survey was pre-tested by volunteers (n=10), average time to answer all questions was approximately nine minutes. Incomplete questionnaires were not accessioned, and response origin IP addresses were monitored to block duplicate submissions. As this research component entailed no direct patient contact or collection of any identifiable personal health information, the study design was considered "no risk to human subjects"; additional IRB oversight was therefore not required.

Statistics

Chi-square test was used for equality of proportions. Maximum likelihood estimation (MLE) was used to determine proportions with 95% confidence interval to assure ≥95% coverage. P-values <0.05 were considered statistically significant. Dispersion of patient age was shown by boxplot among different groups (Frigge *et al.*, 1989).

RESULTS

Valid email contacts were extracted from chart reviews for study patients who completed ovarian PRP during the assessment period (n=188). PRP treatment dates for participants are summarized in Figure 1. From these, full questionnaires were returned by 80 patients (43% response rate). In this sample, mean±SD patient age was 45.5±6 (range = 30.7-63.5, median = 45.1yrs) years. Mean±SD body mass index (BMI) for patients before vs. after PRP was 25±5.1 and 24.7±4.3kg/m^2, respectively. Further analysis of patient weight following ovarian PRP found an average loss of 1kg among study patients (p=0.028).

In this sample, 45 women reported irregular or absent menses at baseline (56.3%); 11 of these (24.4%) observed return of menstruation or resumption of regular menses following ovarian PRP (p=0.041, by binomial proportion z-test). Among 46 women who reported some past or present HRT (hormone replacement therapy) use before enrollment, 31 were able to discontinue HRT following ovarian PRP treatment (67.4%; 95%CI=52%, 80.5%]. There were 11 study patients who were not sexually active before undergoing ovarian PRP. In this subgroup, three women reported resumption of sexual activity after treatment (27.3%). Among patients who were sexually active prior to PRP (n=69), only three women reported negative change in sexual activity after ovarian PRP (4.4%). From these data, it was possible to evaluate reported improvement (27.3%) vs. impairment (4.4%) in sexual activity after ovarian PRP, and this difference was found to be highly significant (p=0.008, by N-1 χ^2 test).

When patients considered their daily average energy level, 45 of 80 patients (56.3%) reported reduced fatigue and beneficial improvement in energy level following ovarian PRP treatment [95%CI=44.7%, 67.3%]. Self-reports were also analyzed for patient observations regarding skin quality, nail growth, and scalp hair thickness/texture after ovarian PRP administration. For these parameters, 37 of 80 patients (46.3%) noted improvement after treatment [95%CI=35%, 57.8%]. Of note, this change following ovarian PRP treatment was found to correlate closely with daily average energy level (Pearson's r=0.41; p<0.001).

Tab. 1. Summary of items assessed by anonymous questionnaire among women who completed intraovarian injection of autologous platelet rich plasma (PRP).

1.	In what year were you born? (enter 4-digit birth year; for example, 1976)
2.	When did you receive PRP at Dr. Sills office?
3.	What is your height in feet and inches?
4.	At the time of your ovarian PRP procedure, what was your approximate weight in pounds?
5.	What is your approximate weight now, in pounds?
6.	Prior to your ovarian PRP treatment, were you having regular (approximately monthly) menses?
7.	Are you having regular (approximately monthly) periods after ovarian PRP, or has your menstrual pattern become more frequent?
8.	Prior to your ovarian PRP treatment, did you ever take prescription HRT (hormone replacement therapy)? Note - this includes birth control pills.
9.	After your ovarian PRP treatment, have you used any prescription HRT (hormone replacement therapy)? Note - this includes birth control pills.
10.	At the time of your ovarian PRP procedure, were you in a relationship which included regular sexual activity?
11.	After ovarian PRP treatment, did you continue your existing intimate relationship OR initiate a new intimate relationship?
12.	Before your ovarian PRP treatment, how would you score your overall energy/activity level?
13.	After your ovarian PRP treatment, how would you score your overall energy/activity level?
14.	Before your ovarian PRP treatment, how would you describe your personal satisfaction with skin, nails, and hair characteristics?
15.	After your ovarian PRP treatment, how would you describe your personal satisfaction with skin, nails, and hair characteristics?
16.	Before your ovarian PRP treatment, how would you score your ability to think clearly (i.e., level of mental/cognitive function)?
17.	After your ovarian PRP treatment, how would you score your ability to think clearly (i.e., level of mental/cognitive function)?
18.	Prior to ovarian PRP treatment, how would you score your ability to get a good night's sleep (i.e., sleep duration & quality)?
19.	Following ovarian PRP treatment, how would you score your ability to get a good night's sleep (i.e., sleep duration & quality)?
	The remaining questions are based on the Female Sexual Function Index (FSFI). In answering these standard queries, the following definitions apply: Sexual activity can include caressing, foreplay, masturbation, and vaginal intercourse. Sexual intercourse is defined as penile penetration (entry) of the vagina. Sexual stimulation includes situations like foreplay, masturbation, or sexual fantasy. Where: 1=almost never, 2=less than half the time, 3=about half the time, 4=more than half the time, 5=almost always.
20.	Before your ovarian PRP procedure, how often did you feel sexual desire or interest?
21.	After your ovarian PRP procedure, how often did you feel sexual desire or interest?
22.	Before your ovarian PRP procedure, how often would you note cervical mucus production or (natural) vaginal lubrication during sexual activity or intercourse?
23.	After your ovarian PRP procedure, how often would you note cervical mucus or (natural) vaginal lubrication during sexual activity or intercourse?
24.	Before your ovarian PRP procedure, how often were you satisfied with your arousal (excitement) during sexual activity or intercourse?
25.	After your ovarian PRP procedure, how often were you satisfied with your arousal (excitement) during sexual activity or intercourse?
26.	Before your ovarian PRP procedure, how often did you reach orgasm (climax) during sexual stimulation?
27.	After your ovarian PRP procedure, how often did you reach orgasm (climax) during sexual stimulation?
28.	Before your ovarian PRP procedure, how often were you satisfied with your overall sexual life?
29.	After your ovarian PRP procedure, how often were you satisfied with your overall sexual life?
30.	Were both of your ovaries able to be accessed and injected with PRP by Dr. Sills (even if this required more than one visit)?

We also sought to measure subjective change in cognitive acuity and mentation after ovarian PRP, and 37 of 80 patients (46.3%) noted increased "clarity of thinking" following the procedure [95%CI=35%, 57.8%]. This reported improvement in cognitive acuity was significantly correlated with both skin improvements (Pearson's r=0.36; p<0.01) and energy level (Pearson's r=0.47; p<0.001). Moreover, overall sleep quality among study subjects was reported to be better by 35 of 80 women (43.8%; 95%CI=32.7%, 55.3%] following ovarian PRP. This significant post-treatment change correlated significantly with skin improvements (Pearson's r=0.42; p<0.01), increased energy level (Pearson's r=0.42; p<0.01), and improved mentation (Pearson's r=0.39; p<0.01).

After ovarian PRP, some study patients observed a substantial change in vaginal lubrication/cervical mucus production; 41 of 80 women indicated these factors had improved (51.3%; 95%CI=39.8%, 62.6%] with significant correlations measured with skin improve-

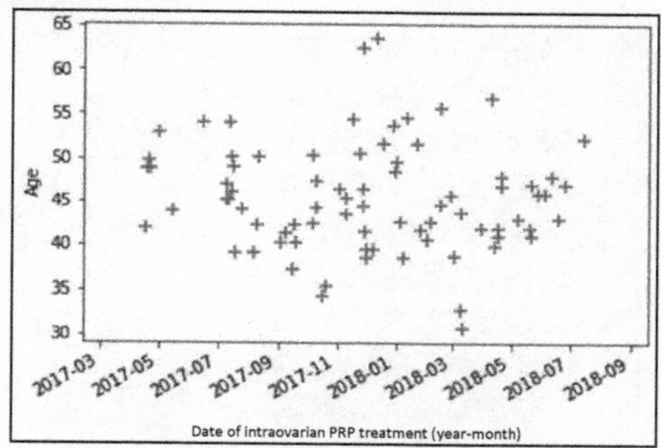

Fig. 1. Distribution of patient age as a function of treatment enrollment date among women (n=80) who completed transvaginal injection of intraovarian PRP.

ments (Pearson's r=0.32; p=0.004), increased energy level (Pearson's r=0.23; p=0.04), improved mentation (Pearson's r=0.28; p=0.011), and improved sleep quality (Pearson's r=0.37; p<0.001).

Moreover, interest in sexual activity was reported as increased by 44 of 80 subjects (55%) [95%CI=43.5%, 66.2%] and this improvement after ovarian PRP was strongly correlated with better skin tone, nail growth, and scalp hair thickness/texture improvements (Pearson's r=0.54; p<0.001), higher energy level (Pearson's r=0.37; p<0.001), clearer thinking/improved mentation (Pearson's r=0.39; p<0.001), as well as better sleep quality (Pearson's r=0.46; p<0.001). A related change in arousal/sexual desire was also noted among study patients following ovarian PRP, such that 37 of 80 women (46.3%; 95%CI=35%, 57.8%) indicated that this was enhanced after treatment, as was the ability to achieve orgasm/climax during sex (45% reported improvement; 95%CI=33.9%, 56.5%). As shown in Figure 2, respondents answering affirmatively regarding improved level of overall sexual experience after ovarian PRP were significantly older than patients who

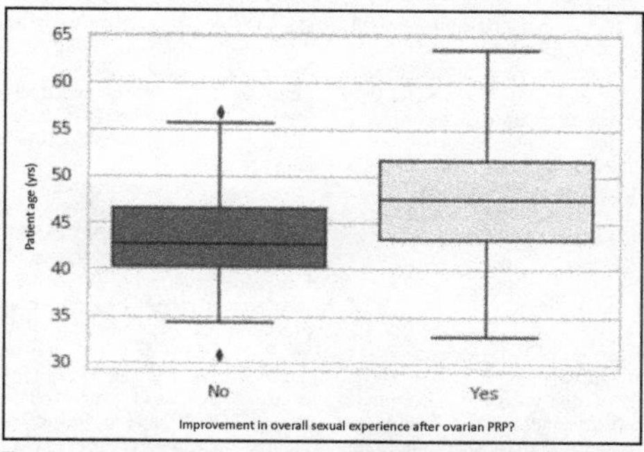

Fig. 2. Improvement of 'overall sexual experience' following intraovarian injection of autologous platelet rich plasma, as measured from anonymous, confidential self reports (n=80). In this sample, mean±SD age for patients responding yes vs. no were 47.9±6.3 vs. 43.5±5.2yrs (p=0.001, by two tailed t-test).

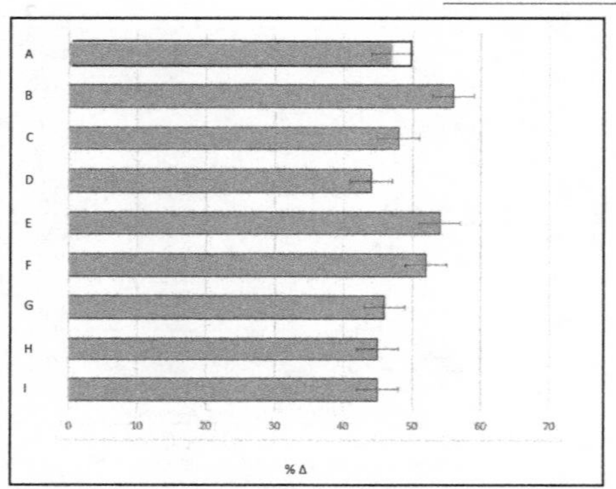

Fig. 3. Change (%Δ) in selected sexual function and metabolic parameters before vs. after intraovarian injection of autologous platelet rich plasma, as measured from anonymous, confidential self reports (n=80). Where: A=skin tone/hair thickness/nail growth, B=daily energy level, C=cognitive clarity, D=sleep quality, E=sexual desire/libido, F=cervical mucus/vaginal lubrication, G=arousal, H=ability to achieve orgasm/climax, I=overall sexual experience.

did not report such change (47.9±6.3 vs. 43.5±5.2yrs; p=0.001). Changes in pre- vs. post-PRP responses across all study parameters are summarized in Figure 3.

Although subjects who enrolled in the RCT usually had both ovaries treated with autologous PRP, this was not possible for 35% of cases (n=28). Unilateral ovarian injection was generally due to limited visibility of adnexal structures via transvaginal ultrasound, secondary to body habitus. Our analysis confirmed that access to one ovary only was significantly correlated to BMI (p=0.027), such that heavier patients were less likely to undergo bilateral ovarian PRP treatment. Nevertheless, sub-analysis of survey data revealed that injection of autologous PRP into just one ovary was similarly effective in manifesting change in overall sex life satisfaction change (p=0.85), energy level (p=0.42), and menses pattern change (p=0.15) compared to bilateral ovarian treatment.

DISCUSSION

Eventual cessation of menses heralds the natural closing of the reproductive window for females (Sills *et al.*, 2009), and the effects of this narrowing therapeutic spectrum in clinical fertility practice often include low ovarian reserve and menstrual irregularity. As a biological process, perimenopause and menopause may be regarded as universal among women of sufficient age, yet the constellation of symptoms can impact productivity and quality of life with much variation (Greening, 2017). Indeed some infertility patients may not confront menopause until many years later, but nevertheless experience features of ovarian ageing—where the challenge of reproductive loss is but one component. Accordingly, fertility issues tend to take the spotlight during IVF consultations while not far from center-stage are equally distressing issues including vaginal discomfort and dryness (Kingsberg & Krychman, 2013; Naumova & Castelo-Branco, 2018), reduced libido (Shifren *et al.*, 2008; Cappelletti & Wallen, 2016), poor sleep quality (Baker *et al.*, 2018; Jones *et al.*, 2018), and cognitive decline (Berent-Spillson *et al.*, 2013; Georgiakis *et al.*, 2016).

Against this background, two publications have discussed ovarian tissue treatment with autologous platelet rich plasma (PRP) specifically as a precursor to *in vitro* fertilization. The initial paper described four poor-prognosis IVF patients (mean age 42yrs) who were consigned to donor oocyte treatment; all produced blastocysts for cryopreservation after ovarian PRP (Sills *et al.*, 2018) and one has since undergone transfer and healthy term delivery. Six months later, researchers in Greece reported on three poor-responder IVF patients (mean age 38yrs) with comparable "revolutionary" outcomes (Sfakianoudis *et al.*, 2018). In the current study, low reserve with irregular or absent menses at baseline was corrected after ovarian PRP in a significant proportion of patients, such that more than half resumed menses and were able to discontinue exogenous hormone replacement therapy (HRT). While the observed changes may or may not be directly connected to follicular recruitment or IVF, we believe they are nevertheless important and deserve closer study.

Prior IVF data on ovarian PRP suggested that leaner women were more likely to respond to this intervention than those with higher BMI (Sills *et al.*, 2018), and the present investigation extends this observation by noting patients lost weight and significantly reduced their BMI (p=0.028) after ovarian PRP. Curiously, while higher BMI was linked to reduced ability to access both ovaries safely for PRP dosing, unilateral ovarian injection did not meaningfully diminish any measured qualitative outcome.

While estradiol and testosterone are both ovarian products important in modulating female sexual and neurobehavioral response (Dhanuka & Simon, 2015; Cappelletti & Wallen, 2016; Fantasia, 2016), how these sex steroids might be affected by injection of PRP into the ovary is not known. Of note, significant increases in sexual activity, improved ability to reach orgasm/climax, and better overall sexual experience were reported following ovarian PRP injection here. It is plausible that a higher level of ovarian endocrine output results from autologous PRP "rescue", explaining why our patients reported significant improvements in sleep quality, energy level, dermatological characteristics like nails/skin/scalp hair, clarity of thinking, as well as cervical mucus production and vaginal lubrication. The finding of improved overall sexual experience among patients at significantly higher age (vs. non-responders) invites additional study and suggests ovaries in such older women could be more sensitive to or better suited for ovarian PRP.

Based on the scope of changes experienced by these patients, should ovarian PRP be considered for symptomatic women not necessarily aspiring to retrieve their own eggs? A growing body of literature now addresses ovarian senescence, usually with emphasis on lifestyle modification, calorie restriction, toxin avoidance, and especially pharmacologic interventions like assorted HRT regimes. Because symptoms can sometimes be severe and refractory, multiple strategies are often deployed simultaneously with varying efficacy. If our results can be validated by additional multicenter studies, ovarian treatment with autologous PRP could join these interventions and become a useful therapeutic addition—not just as an antecedent to IVF as initially proposed (Sfakianoudis *et al.*, 2018; Sills *et al.*, 2018) but for general management of systemic perimenopausal symptoms.

How might the dramatic changes observed here be explained? What is it about injecting autologous PRP into ovarian tissue—considered impaired or dormant in most cases—that could yield an apparent alteration in function? Discussion of IVF cycle data after ovarian PRP permitted some conjecture (Sills *et al.*, 2018), and the findings reported here appear to point in the same direction. Specifically, administration of activated PRP delivers growth factors, chemokines, and cytokines such as stromal cell derived factor-1 and hepatocyte growth factor deep into ovarian tissue. Upon arrival these and other molecular signals orchestrate tissue perfusion and angiogenesis (Szafarowska & Jerzak, 2013), possibly setting the stage for ovarian re-potentiation. Indeed, placement of these PRP-derived cell signals might "switch on" adult ovaries with low or absent reserve by establishing communication channels with uncommitted ovarian stem cells, thus creating local signaling contexts to induce differentiation towards (hormonally) active follicles. As proposed earlier (Sfakianoudis *et al.*, 2018; Sills *et al.* 2018), this sequence could also entail postnatal oogenesis - a pathbreaking but unsettled principle for fertility practice where research both in support (Virant-Klun *et al.*, 2012; Woods *et al.*, 2013) and in opposition (Byskov *et al.*, 2011; Zhang *et al.*, 2012) exists.

Several limitations of our work should be acknowledged. Any questionnaire used to collect *post hoc* data could be subject to recall bias among respondents. Here the interval between PRP intervention and clinical assessment was limited, and this method has been successfully applied to assess sexual response after other gynecology procedures (Saini *et al.*, 2002). In addition, it would have been ideal to have captured more detail on quality of life changes over time, especially about which changes were experienced in what sequence (and duration of their effects), although this awaits further longitudinal study in larger populations. Finally, our analysis would have been substantially strengthened if the qualitative changes reported privately here were linked on a case-by-case basis to laboratory data collected after ovarian PRP. These data do exist and form the basis of further investigations, but to preserve patient confidentiality our anonymous survey could not make that connection.

In summary, while ovarian injection with autologous PRP has achieved significantly improved reserve markers (Sills *et al.*, 2018) and yielded livebirths from poor prognosis IVF patients using their own oocytes (Sfakianoudis *et al.*, 2018), the neurobehavioral and metabolic changes measured here position ovarian PRP beyond conventional fertility practice. Here, we offer evidence of improvement in multiple quality of life parameters following use of intraovarian PRP. To clarify which patient characteristics may predict responsiveness to ovarian PRP, as well as how best to refine this minimally invasive technique, additional clinical research is underway.

CONFLICT OF INTEREST DISCLOSURE

ESS holds a provisional U.S. patent for process & treatment using ovarian platelet rich plasma.

REFERENCES

1 Baker FC, Lampio L, Saaresranta T et al. (2018). Sleep and Sleep Disorders in the Menopausal Transition. Sleep Med Clin **13**(3): 443-56.
2 Berent-Spillson A, Briceno E, Pinsky A et al. (2015). Distinct cognitive effects of estrogen and progesterone in menopausal women. Psychoneuroendocrinology **59**:25-36.
3 Byskov AG, Hoyer PE, Andersen CY et al. (2011). No evidence for the presence of oogonia in the human ovary after their final clearance during the first two years of life. Hum Reprod **26**:2129–39.
4 Cappelletti M, Wallen K (2016). Increasing women's sexual desire: The comparative effectiveness of estrogens and androgens. Horm Behav **78**: 178-93.
5 Crisp CC, Fellner AN, Pauls RN (2015). Validation of the Female Sexual Function Index (FSFI) for web-based administration. Int Urogynecol J. **26**(2): 219-22.
6 Dhanuka I, Simon JA (2015). Flibanserin for the treatment of hypoactive sexual desire disorder in premenopausal women. Expert Opin Pharmacother. **16**(16): 2523-9.
7 Fantasia HC (2016). Flibanserin and Female Sexual Desire. Nurs Womens Health. **20**(3): 309-14.
8 Frigge M, Hoaglin DC, Iglewicz B (1989). Some implementations of the boxplot. Am Stat **43**: 50-4.
9 Georgakis MK, Kalogirou EI, Diamantaras AA et al. (2016). Age at menopause and duration of reproductive period in association with dementia and cognitive function: A systematic review and meta-analysis. Psychoneuroendocrinology **73**: 224-43.
10 Greening J (2017). Menopause transition: effects on women's economic participation. HM Government Equalities Office [United Kingdom]; July 20, 2017: https://www.gov.uk/government/publications/menopause-transition-effects-on-womens-economic-participation [site accessed August 20, 2018].
11 Gurtner GC, Werner S, Barrandon Y et al. (2008). Wound repair and regeneration. Nature. **453**: 314–21.
12 Jones HJ, Zak R, Lee KA (2018). Sleep Disturbances in Midlife Women at the Cusp of the Menopausal Transition. J Clin Sleep Med **14**(7): 1127-33.
13 Kingsberg SA, Krychman ML (2013). Resistance and barriers to local estrogen therapy in women with atrophic vaginitis. J Sex Med **10**(6): 1567-74.
14 Lacci KM, Dardik A (2010). Platelet-rich plasma: support for its use in wound healing. Yale J Biol Med **83**: 1–9.
15 Naumova I, Castelo-Branco C (2018). Current treatment options for postmenopausal vaginal atrophy. Int J Womens Health **10**: 387-395.
16 Nurden AT (2011). Platelets, inflammation and tissue regeneration. Thromb Haemost **105**(Suppl.1): S13–S33.
17 Saini J, Kuczynski E, Gretz HF 3rd et al. (2002). Supracervical hysterectomy versus total abdominal hysterectomy: perceived effects on sexual function. BMC Womens Health **2**(1): 1.
18 Sfakianoudis K, Simopoulou M, Nitsos N et al. (2018). A Case Series on Platelet-Rich Plasma Revolutionary Management of Poor Responder Patients. Gynecol Obstet Invest 2018: 1-8 doi: 10.1159/000491697.
19 Shifren JL, Monz BU, Russo PA et al. (2008). Sexual problems and distress in United States women: Prevalence and correlates. Obstet Gynecol **112**(5): 970–8.
20 Sills ES, Alper MM, Walsh AP (2009). Ovarian reserve screening in infertility: practical applications and theoretical directions for research. Eur J Obstet Gynecol Reprod Biol **146**(1): 30-6.
21 Sills ES, Rickers NS, Li X et al. (2018). First data on in vitro fertilization and blastocyst formation after intraovarian injection of calcium gluconate-activated autologous platelet rich plasma. Gynecol Endocrinol **28**: 1-5.
22 Szafarowska M, Jerzak M (2013). Ovarian aging and infertility. Ginekol Pol **84**: 298–304.
23 U.S. National Library of Medicine (2017). Autologous platelet-rich plasma (PRP) infusions and biomarkers of ovarian rejuvenation and ageing mitigation (NCT03178695); March 7, 2017 https://clinicaltrials.gov/ct2/show/study/NCT03178695 [site accessed August 20, 2018].
24 Virant-Klun I, Stimpfel M, Skutella T (2012). Stem cells in adult human ovaries: from female fertility to ovarian cancer. Curr Pharm Des **18**: 283–92.
25 Woods DC, White YA, Tilly JL (2013). Purification of oogonial stem cells from adult mouse and human ovaries: an assessment of the literature and a view toward the future. Reprod Sci **20**: 7–15.
26 Zhang H, Zheng W, Shen Y et al. (2012). Experimental evidence showing that no mitotically active female germline progenitors exist in postnatal mouse ovaries. Proc Natl Acad Sci USA **109**: 12580–5.

CPSIA information can be obtained
at www.ICGtesting.com
Printed in the USA
BVHW072354120819
555662BV00008B/1191/P